Bold Women in History

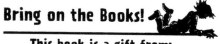

Bold Women
IN HISTORY

15 WOMEN'S RIGHTS ACTIVISTS
YOU SHOULD KNOW

Meghan Vestal

Illustrated by Keisha Morris

ROCKRIDGE
PRESS

For general information on our other products and services or to obtain technical support, please contact our Customer Care Department within the United States at (866) 744-2665, or outside the United States at (510) 253-0500.

Rockridge Press publishes its books in a variety of electronic and print formats. Some content that appears in print may not be available in electronic books, and vice versa.

Series Designer: William Mack
Interior and Cover Designer: Heather Krakora
Art Producer: Hannah Dickerson
Editor: Barbara J. Isenberg
Production Editor: Andrew Yackira
Production Manager: Jose Olivera

Illustrations © 2021 Keisha Morris
Decorative pattern used under license from Shutterstock.com
Author photo courtesy of Ben Vestal Online
Illustrator photo courtesy of Emma Wynn Paul

ISBN: Print 978-1-64876-429-5 | eBook 978-1-64876-430-1
R0

Thank you to my grandmothers, Doris and Shirley. They taught me how to think independently, stand up for what is right, lead in the workplace, and love family. I would not be the person I am today without their examples.

Contents

Introduction viii

Elizabeth Cady STANTON 1

Susan B. ANTHONY 9

Sojourner TRUTH 15

Frances Ellen Watkins HARPER 21

Ida B. WELLS-BARNETT 27

Marie Louise Bottineau BALDWIN 33

Mary McLeod BETHUNE 39

Adelina "Nina" OTERO-WARREN 45

Alice PAUL 51

Mabel PING-HUA LEE 57

Betty FRIEDAN 63

Ruth Bader GINSBURG 69

Gloria STEINEM 75

bell hooks 81

Stacey ABRAMS 87

Glossary 92

References 95

Introduction

What do you want to be when you grow up? You have so many options. You can become a doctor, manage a major corporation, or even run for president! Just 150 years ago, none of these things would have been possible because the voices of women were silenced in most aspects of American life.

Then in the late 19th century, a group of women decided they would be silenced no more. Lucretia Mott, Elizabeth Cady Stanton, and Susan B. Anthony started the women's suffrage **movement**, which was the first women's rights movement in the United States. "Suffrage" means the right to vote. Suffragists, or people who worked for suffrage, spent more than 70 years leading protests and parades, demanding that women be given a voice in political elections. Many of the suffragists were called names, spit on, and imprisoned. They made these sacrifices so that you and all women could have a voice in elections.

Even after the 19th Amendment of the Constitution gave women the right to vote, there was still work to be done. A woman was still viewed as a second-class **citizen** and did not have a voice in higher education or the work-place. Most women did not work. They were expected to stay home with their children, whether they wanted to or not. Those who tried to work were prevented from taking high-ranking jobs or were fired if they became pregnant.

In the 1960s, women such as Angela Davis, Dolores Huerta, Audre Lorde, Betty Friedan, and Gloria Steinem started a new women's liberation movement, known as the **feminist** movement. The feminist movement sought to give women **equality** in all aspects of American life, especially the workplace. Thanks to feminists, women now make up more than 50 percent of college graduates each year. Women are also now recognized as valuable members of the workforce. Many women are CEOs and government leaders.

Even though the women that led these movements lived at different times and fought for different issues, they all had one thing in common. They were not working only for themselves. They were working to give future generations of women a voice, too.

Prepare to journey alongside 15 bold women who impacted the lives of all American women. Throughout the journey, you'll meet Alice Paul, who was imprisoned and tortured for promoting women's suffrage. You'll also meet Mary McLeod Bethune, who fought to ensure all women had access to education and the polls, even when hate groups tried to stop it. Then you'll meet Mabel Ping-Hua Lee, who dedicated her early life to women's suffrage even though she knew she would not receive voting rights if a suffrage amendment was passed.

As you approach the end of this book, you'll realize that this is just the beginning of your journey. Women such as bell hooks and Stacey Abrams are still fighting for equality at the polls, the workplace, and in education. And there are many more important women in history who could not be included in this book. This book is just a starting point. As you read about each of these bold women, I hope you feel inspired to pick up the torch and use your voice to advocate for equality. Just as these women have paved the way for the opportunities you have today, you can continue to pave the way for future generations of women.

Let the journey begin!

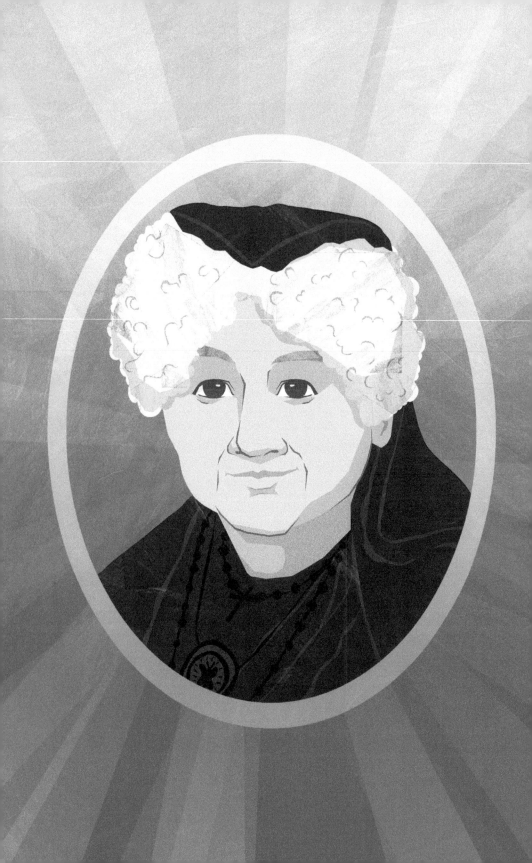

Elizabeth Cady
STANTON

1815–1902

Have you ever considered how a movement to spark change begins? Movements like women's suffrage didn't just happen. They began because brave individuals made the choice to stand up for what was right, no matter the cost. Elizabeth Cady Stanton was a spark that started the women's suffrage movement.

Elizabeth was born into one of the wealthiest families in Johnston, New York. Being born into a life of privilege allowed Elizabeth to attend some of the best schools for women. Elizabeth enjoyed reading and writing. She would even study in her father's law office and read his legal books. It was there that Elizabeth read about laws and **discrimination** against women.

These laws angered her, and she wanted to fight them. The problem was that, at the time, there weren't any large groups working together for women's rights. Someone would have to start the first group. It would take several years before Elizabeth became that person.

Elizabeth's **activist** career started with the anti-slavery movement. Elizabeth's parents wanted her to keep her political ideas to herself. She defied their wishes and married an **abolitionist** speaker. She worked alongside her husband to protest slavery. It was while working with her husband in 1840 that Elizabeth's life took a turn and she began to step into the spotlight.

In 1840, Elizabeth and her husband were in London for the World Anti-Slavery Convention. Thousands of people came to hear abolitionists speak about the curse of slavery. But Elizabeth was banned from attending the convention. The leaders of the equal rights movement refused to let women in. Elizabeth and her friends were frustrated, but they had an idea. They would start a women's rights movement in the United States!

When Elizabeth returned from London, she began working to draw more attention to women's issues such as voting rights and property rights. Movements typically don't succeed without a large following. Elizabeth knew that she would have to bring attention to the cause to help it grow. She planned the first women's rights convention. The convention would raise awareness by defining and sharing the message of the women's suffrage movement.

In 1848, 300 people attended the Seneca Falls Convention. During the two-day meeting, Elizabeth helped write the Declaration of Sentiments. The document revised the Declaration of Independence by adding that "all men *and women* are created equal." The declaration also listed 19 things that women wanted changed. They included the lack of voting rights, the inability to own property, and unequal wages to men. The document is often credited as the start of the women's rights movement.

> **"WE HOLD THESE TRUTHS TO BE SELF-EVIDENT: THAT ALL MEN AND WOMEN ARE CREATED EQUAL."**

Soon after the convention, Elizabeth met Susan B. Anthony (page 9). During the 1850s, it was tough for Elizabeth to travel because she had seven young children. So, Elizabeth wrote speeches about women's rights. Then Susan traveled the country to deliver the speeches.

During the Civil War, Elizabeth paused her work in the women's suffrage movement to assist with the anti-slavery movement. In 1863, Elizabeth and Susan started the Women's National Loyal League. The organization worked to end the war through a constitutional amendment to abolish slavery. More than 5,000 women joined the league, agreeing to pause their work in the women's suffrage movement to help people of color secure freedom.

The league received national recognition for starting an anti-slavery petition that was signed by more than

400,000 people. In 1865, the 13th Amendment was ratified, officially abolishing slavery in the United States. After the amendment passed, the league dissolved and the women returned to fighting for women's rights.

Even though Elizabeth supported equal rights for all, she was outraged by the 15th Amendment, which gave Black men, but not women, the right to vote. The amendment created a division in the women's suffrage movement. Most suffragists saw it as a stepping-stone for women gaining the right to vote. Elizabeth did not think the amendment should have passed without saying that women were also citizens who could vote.

The disagreement between suffragists led Elizabeth and Susan to form a new organization for women, the National Woman Suffrage Association (NWSA). Elizabeth served as the president. The NWSA worked to bring women's suffrage to the attention of government leaders and the public.

In 1878, Elizabeth helped write a federal suffrage amendment giving women the right to vote. The amendment was proposed in Congress every year between 1878 and 1919. Members of the NWSA would travel to Washington, DC, to speak before leaders at the capitol. Elizabeth spoke in Congress many times, and she was always shocked by how the congressmen behaved. They ignored women as they spoke and read newspapers instead.

Elizabeth spent her later years writing. She worked with Susan on *History of Woman Suffrage*, a book that tells the story of the women's suffrage movement. Elizabeth also wrote *The Woman's Bible*, in which she stated that men used religion to limit women's rights. Elizabeth was criticized for her claims, even by other suffragists. Her final book was *Eighty Years and More*, an autobiography. People still read Elizabeth's books today. Her writings help modern Americans better understand women's suffrage and what many women sacrificed to help future generations of women.

Elizabeth died in 1902. She did not live to see women vote, but her work affected all future generations of American women. Women would have never received the right to vote if someone hadn't been willing to step forward and organize the women's suffrage movement. In beginning the conversation about women's suffrage, Elizabeth inspired more women to take action and demand equality.

EXPLORE MORE! Elizabeth Cady Stanton wrote many speeches throughout her life. You can examine her handwritten speeches on the Library of Congress website at LOC.gov. (Enter "Elizabeth Cady Stanton papers" in the search box.)

DID YOU KNOW? There used to be one organization that sought equal rights for all people: the American

Equal Rights Association (AERA). When the 15th Amendment created disagreement between suffragists, the AERA women divided into two new organizations: the National Woman Suffrage Association and the American Woman Suffrage Association. The organizations worked separately for the same cause. In 1890, the organizations merged into the National American Woman Suffrage Association (NAWSA). Elizabeth served as the president of the NAWSA.

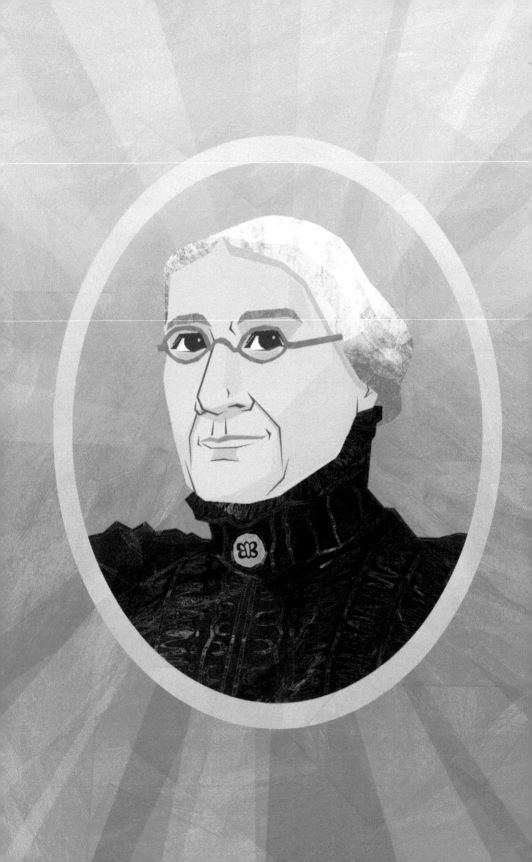

Susan B. ANTHONY
1820–1906

Some might say Susan B. Anthony was born with activism in her blood. As a child, she watched her parents and siblings fight for equal rights for all people. As an adult, she joined the fight for equality, becoming one of the most well-known leaders of the women's suffrage movement.

Susan and her family were Quakers. The Quaker faith teaches that all people are created equal. As a result of this belief, Susan's family supported the abolition of slavery. During Susan's early years, the family's home was a meeting place for abolitionists. The famous abolitionist Frederick Douglass was even a frequent visitor in their home. Frederick had escaped slavery. He gained worldwide fame after publishing an autobiography about being enslaved.

Much of Susan's early work supported the abolition of slavery. Knowing Frederick and hearing his stories inspired Susan to get involved. In the 19th century, people thought it was wrong for women to give speeches or openly discuss politics. That didn't stop Susan. She used her skill as a speaker to share the need for racial equality.

Susan's parents not only worked to abolish slavery. Her mother and sister were also early supporters of the women's suffrage movement. They attended women's rights conventions and openly worked to help women secure the right to vote. This brought women's rights to Susan's attention at a young age, although she did not get heavily involved in the women's suffrage movement until after 1851.

> "IF I COULD LIVE ANOTHER CENTURY! I DO SO WANT TO SEE THE FRUITION OF THE WORK FOR WOMEN IN THE PAST CENTURY. THERE IS SO MUCH YET TO BE DONE, I SEE SO MANY THINGS I WOULD LIKE TO DO AND SAY, BUT I MUST LEAVE IT FOR THE YOUNGER GENERATION."

In 1851, Susan attended an anti-slavery convention in New York. There, Susan met an early leader of women's suffrage, Elizabeth Cady Stanton (page 1). The women became great friends. It was after that meeting that Susan became more involved in the women's suffrage movement, and it took a priority in her life. Susan and Elizabeth spent more than 50 years fighting for women's rights together by giving speeches, writing articles and books, organizing events, and founding equal rights organizations.

The fight for equality wasn't easy. The 14th Amendment, which was ratified, or passed, in 1868, defined a citizen as "all persons born or naturalized in the United States" and granted all citizens equal protection under the law. A few years later, the 15th Amendment gave citizens the right to vote, regardless of color.

That constitutional definition of a citizen did not specify gender. So, Susan decided to test the amendments. In 1872, she voted in New York. Shortly after, a police officer appeared at her house and arrested her. A trial was set for a few weeks after her arrest. In the weeks leading up to the trial, Susan traveled throughout New York. She shared her story with crowds of people and raised the question: Is it a crime for a US citizen to vote?

When it came time for the trial, the judge refused to allow the jury to hear testimonies or view evidence. He ordered the jury to find Susan guilty. Susan was fined $100 for voting. She did not pay the fine.

In the years that followed, Susan worked tirelessly for women's right to vote. She knew that receiving the right to vote would open doors for women in all areas of life. If women could elect their leaders, they could vote for people who would support women's issues. Susan gave speeches across the country, published books about the history of women's suffrage, and produced a newspaper about women's issues. All of these things helped bring attention to the movement.

Later, in 1900, the University of Rochester was forced to accept female students for the first time, thanks to Susan. When the university would not admit women due to cost, Susan raised more than $50,000 to ensure women could receive an education. She also helped get the Nurse Practice Act passed in 1903, which provided more education and training for nurses.

In 1905, Susan met with President Theodore Roosevelt. She asked the president to help pass a women's suffrage amendment in Congress. President Roosevelt did not see a need for the amendment at the time, but the meeting had a lasting impact. After his presidency, in 1912, he became a supporter of and activist for the women's suffrage movement.

Like the encounter with President Roosevelt, Susan's work was crucial in laying the groundwork for what was to come. The 19th Amendment finally passed in 1920, giving women the right to vote. Susan was never able to legally vote herself because the amendment passed 14 years after she died.

Many people associate Susan only with women's suffrage. But Susan dedicated her life to fighting for greater equality overall, including labor rights and educational rights. In 1860, Susan used her voice to help pass the New York State Married Women's Property Bill. At the time, a married woman could not own anything. All property belonged to her husband. If a woman worked, her wages were her husband's property. The bill let married women own property and keep their wages.

Today, the US government looks very different, thanks to Susan. In the years that followed the passage of the 19th Amendment, more women were elected to all levels of government. Laws were also passed that increased women's rights in the workplace and gave women more access to education and healthcare. Since the 1980s, women have consistently turned out to vote in higher numbers than men in presidential elections, meaning the voices of women are louder than ever before.

EXPLORE MORE! Want to learn about Susan? Visit the National Susan B. Anthony Museum and House in Rochester, New York, or online at SusanB.org.

DID YOU KNOW? In 1875, the Supreme Court ruled that women are "citizens." But the court also stated that citizens were not entitled to vote. The decision of whether women could vote was left up to the state governments. With this ruling, all American women would only receive the right to vote if a constitutional amendment was passed.

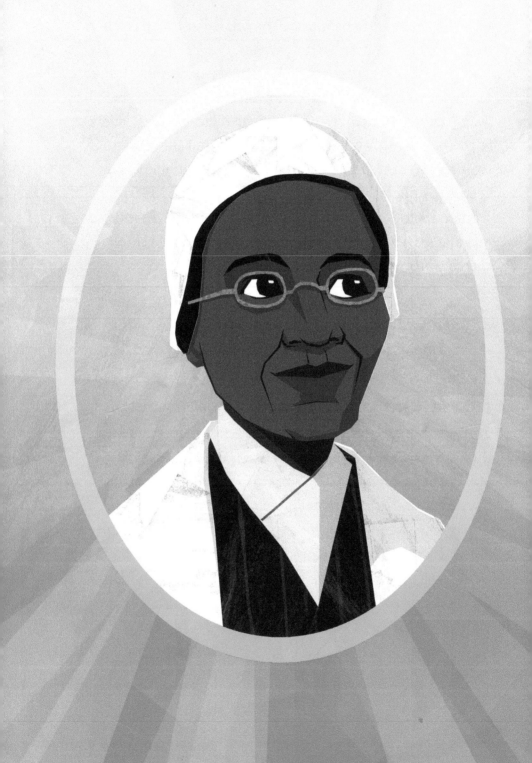

Sojourner TRUTH

1797–1883

How does an enslaved woman who is unable to read or write become a best-selling author and nationally recognized speaker? Given her background, it may have seemed impossible for Sojourner Truth to become one of the leading equal rights activists of her time. But she never allowed what she could not do stop her from helping others.

Isabella Baumfree was born into slavery in New York in 1797. She was separated from her parents as a child after being sold to a different farm. Each day, she was required to perform physically tough jobs and was regularly beaten by her enslavers.

Isabella was forbidden from marrying the man she loved because he was enslaved on another farm. Instead, she was forced to marry an enslaved man on the farm where she lived. She had five children. Fighting for her children's freedom led Isabella to join the anti-slavery movement later in life.

Isabella's enslaver promised to free her in 1826. When the time came, he changed his mind and refused to let her go. Isabella ran away to a nearby abolitionist home. Her enslaver followed and demanded that she be returned. The abolitionists refused to send Isabella back to a life of slavery. They bought her services and gave Isabella her freedom.

Isabella was not content to sit around and enjoy her newfound freedom. She discovered one of her sons had been sold to a farm in Alabama. It was illegal to sell enslaved people across state lines, so she took the enslaver to court and won, retaking custody of her son. Isabella was the first Black woman to sue a white man and win. Soon after, all of her children were freed when slavery was abolished in New York in 1828.

Isabella became an active member of the Christian community in New York, attending religious revivals and speaking at church events. In 1843, she declared that God had told her to preach the truth throughout the country. After the revelation, she changed her name to Sojourner Truth and became a traveling preacher.

Sojourner's career as an equal rights activist began after moving to the Northampton Association of Education and Industry, a religious community in Massachusetts. Many famous abolitionists were a part of the community, including Frederick Douglass. Frederick encouraged Sojourner to become more involved in the anti-slavery movement. She spent many months each year traveling the country and sharing stories from her life.

In 1850, she dictated her biography. Sojourner never learned to read or write, so she had someone write her story for her. *The Narrative of Sojourner Truth* was a huge success. For many, reading Sojourner's book was the first time they had ever heard about the horrors of slavery. Sojourner was able to live off her book sales and use the profits to fund her speaking tours. The book is still sold today and continues to educate readers about the wrongs of slavery.

> **"NOW, IF YOU WANT ME TO GET OUT OF THE WORLD, YOU HAD BETTER GET THE WOMEN VOTIN' SOON. I SHAN'T GO TILL I CAN DO THAT."**

Sojourner's mission to spread truth also included sharing the message of gender equality. She became an outspoken voice in the women's suffrage movement. In 1851, she attended the Ohio Women's Rights Convention, where she gave one of her most famous speeches, "Ain't I a Woman?" She demanded equality for women, including women of color. In the 1850s, it was controversial for women to publicly speak about suffrage, especially women of color. But Sojourner spoke so powerfully and made her point so clearly that some thought she was a man.

Sojourner spent decades traveling and giving speeches about equality. She was accused of being a man because of her excellent speaking abilities on more than one occasion. She became tired of the accusation and unbuttoned her top at one event to prove she was a woman!

Sojourner's involvement in the women's suffrage movement created tension with other anti-slavery leaders, including her friend Frederick. While the abolitionist leaders supported equality for women, too, many believed Black men should receive the right to vote first. Sojourner refused to support a voting rights amendment to the Constitution unless it included all people.

Sojourner's books and speaking events made her a well-known equal rights activist throughout the United States. Even President Abraham Lincoln was impressed by her work. In 1864, President Lincoln invited her to the White House. At the historic meeting, she shared her vision for gender and racial equality. This was one of the first times a woman of color was invited to the White House by a president.

Sojourner continued traveling the country and speaking her truth until she died in 1883. Despite their disagreement over voting rights, Frederick gave a speech at her funeral. He said, "She has been for the last 40 years an object of respect and admiration to social reformers everywhere."

Since her passing, more than 10 memorials have been erected in her honor. She has also been included on the Smithsonian's list of "100 Most Significant Americans" and had a US postage stamp with her picture on it. Today,

Sojourner continues to serve as a model for equal rights activists. Many reformers look to her example of unwavering commitment to the movements she fought for.

EXPLORE MORE! Decide what Sojourner actually said in her "Ain't I a Woman" speech. The Sojourner Truth Project was created to compile and compare different accounts of the famous speech. You can compare speeches by visiting TheSojournerTruthProject.com.

DID YOU KNOW? The phrase "ain't I a woman" may have not have been part of the famous "Ain't I a Woman" speech. Twelve years after presenting the speech, the transcript was published by a person who was at the women's rights convention. Later, other transcripts were published. Each transcript is different, and only the first used the phrase "ain't I a woman." Historians believe the phrase likely was not used because Sojourner was from New York and did not speak using a Southern dialect.

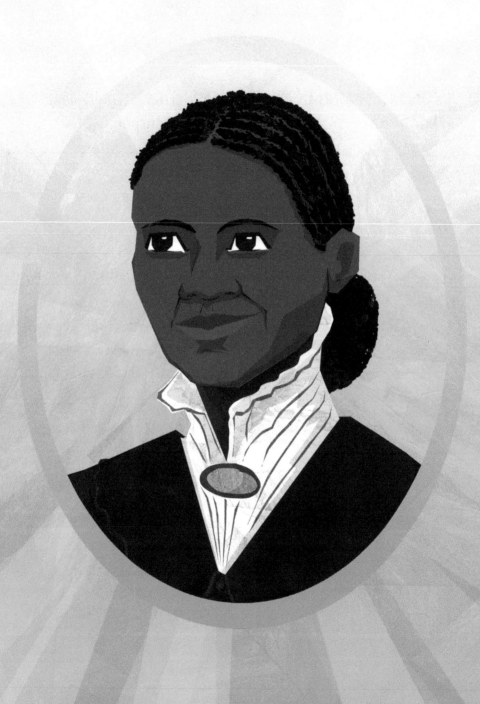

Frances Ellen Watkins
HARPER
1825–1911

Frances Ellen Watkins Harper accomplished many firsts. She was the first Black American woman to publish a short story and the first woman to teach at a certain Ohio school. Of all her accomplishments, Frances's work in the anti-slavery and women's suffrage movements were what she was most proud of.

Frances was born to free Black American parents in Maryland in 1825. Both of her parents died by the time Frances was three years old, and she was raised by her aunt and uncle. Frances's uncle was an abolitionist who started a school for Black children. Frances attended her uncle's school, where she discovered her love of reading and writing poetry. Some of her poems were even published in abolitionist newspapers.

In the 19th century, not all girls could attend school, especially girls of color. Frances recognized how special it was to be educated. She became a teacher so that she could help educate other young girls. She moved to Ohio, where she became the first woman to teach at

Union Theological Seminary. Frances was not warmly welcomed because of her gender. So, after a year, she transferred to a school in Pennsylvania.

While in Pennsylvania, the state of Maryland passed a new slavery law. The law stated that any Black Americans who entered Maryland through the northern border could be imprisoned and sold into slavery. The law prevented Frances from returning home. Even though she was a free woman, she risked being enslaved if she tried to visit her family. This sparked Frances's interest in the anti-slavery movement.

> **"WE ARE ALL BOUND UP TOGETHER IN ONE GREAT BUNDLE OF HUMANITY, AND SOCIETY CANNOT TRAMPLE ON THE WEAKEST AND FEEBLEST OF ITS MEMBERS WITHOUT RECEIVING THE CURSE IN ITS OWN SOUL."**

Soon after, Frances moved in with William and Letitia Still. William was known as the "father of the Underground Railroad." Frances became involved with the Underground Railroad, a secret network used to help enslaved Black Americans escape the South and find freedom in the North. She also traveled throughout the northern states, giving speeches against slavery. Frances often incorporated her love for poetry into her speeches and used poetry to discuss issues related to equality.

In addition to her speaking tours, Frances published two poetry books by 1854. Thousands of copies were sold throughout the United States. Frances donated a large portion of her book earnings to the Underground Railroad.

When traveling, Frances also spoke about issues related to women's rights and became involved in the women's suffrage movement. In 1859, she became the first Black woman in the United States to publish a short story when "The Two Offers" was printed in a magazine. "The Two Offers" told a story about two women who consider two marriage proposals, and it shed light on the limited rights of women at the time. The story was a success and helped promote Frances as a women's suffrage leader.

Not all suffragists supported Frances. While some praised her work and involvement in the women's rights movement, others thought the color of her skin would prevent women from getting the vote in Southern states. In 1866, Frances gave her famous "We Are All Bound Up Together" speech at the National Woman's Rights Convention, where she encouraged her fellow suffragists to include Black women in the movement. The audience did not want to consider this notion. Many women still refused to welcome Black Americans into the movement.

After the 15th Amendment was ratified in 1870, giving Black men the right to vote, a divide grew within the women's suffrage movement. White suffragists such as

Susan B. Anthony and Elizabeth Cady Stanton opposed the 15th Amendment. They believed an amendment should only be passed if it included women. Frances supported the amendment, seeing it as a stepping-stone to women receiving the right to vote.

The divide led to the formation of multiple women's suffrage organizations. Susan and Elizabeth formed the National Woman Suffrage Association (NWSA). Frances joined other men and women who supported the 15th Amendment in the American Woman Suffrage Association (AWSA).

There were many key differences between the NWSA and AWSA. In addition to supporting the 15th Amendment, the AWSA focused solely on women's suffrage and encouraged male involvement in the movement. The NWSA fought for many issues related to women's rights and did not welcome men. Eventually, the groups decided it was better to work together and merged in 1890, forming the National American Woman Suffrage Association (NAWSA).

Frances continued to fight for equal rights for Black women throughout the rest of her life. In 1896, she helped found the National Association of Colored Women's Clubs (NACWC) with other Black **civil rights** leaders, including Harriet Tubman and Ida B. Wells-Barnett (page 27). The organization promoted causes important to Black women, including suffrage, education, and healthcare. By 1924, the NACWC had more than 100,000 members.

Frances did not work as much during the last few years of her life, but always made time to support women's suffrage and the NACWC before she died in 1911. Today, Frances's writing is still highly recognized for its significance in both the anti-slavery and women's suffrage movements. Her writings not only provide modern Americans insight into these movements, but also help people better understand the hardships faced by Black women in the 19th century.

EXPLORE MORE! Frances was nationally recognized for her poetry. You can find and read many of her poems on Poets.org. (Enter "Frances Ellen Watkins Harper" in the search box.)

DID YOU KNOW? When Frances was born, Maryland was a slave state. Slavery was not abolished in Maryland until 1864. Until that time, most Black Americans were enslaved, but there was a small number of free Black Americans living in Maryland. Free Black Americans did not have the same rights as white people. They had to carry proof of their freedom at all times in case they were stopped and questioned.

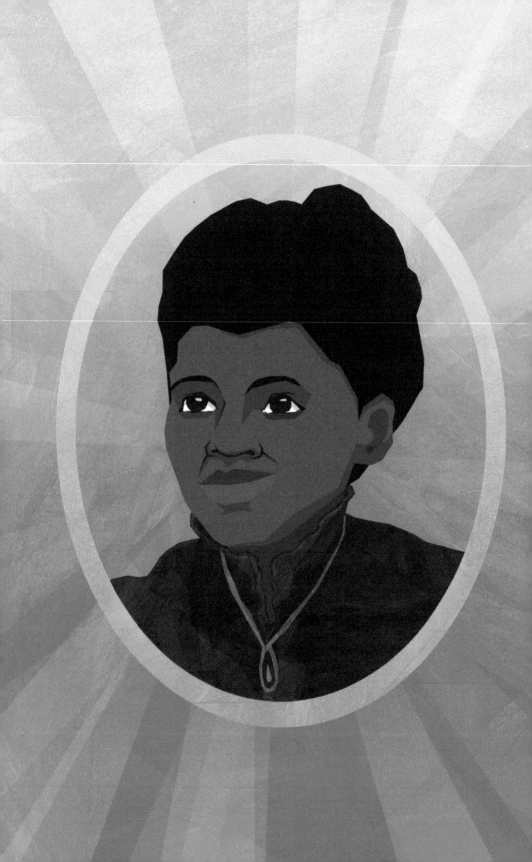

Ida B.
WELLS-BARNETT
1862–1931

Muckrakers were journalists who exposed, or uncovered, corruption at the start of the 20th century. Most were men who wanted to expose politicians and corporations. But there was one woman who used muckraking to expose American **racism**. Ida B. Wells-Barnett exposed the reality of racism in many areas of life, including the women's suffrage movement.

Ida was born into slavery during the Civil War. As enslaved people, Ida's parents were not allowed to read or write. They wanted Ida to have opportunities they didn't have and encouraged her to get an education after the war ended and slavery was abolished. When Ida was 16 years old, yellow fever killed her parents. She moved to Memphis, Tennessee, and took a job as a teacher to support her siblings.

In 1884, an event changed Ida's life forever. She was forcibly removed from a first-class train car even though she had paid for a ticket. As the railroad workers dragged her off the train, white passengers applauded. Ida sued the railroad company. She won, but a higher court overturned the decision. The press gave the case a lot of attention. Many were amazed that a young Black woman would stand up to a large company. Ida's interviews with the press sparked her interest in journalism.

> ## "THE WAY TO RIGHT WRONGS IS TO TURN THE LIGHT OF TRUTH UPON THEM."

Shortly after, Ida became part owner of the *Memphis Free Speech* newspaper. She used the newspaper to speak out against racism. In 1892, Ida published her first major story. Three Black men had opened a market that was taking customers away from a white-owned market. One night, people broke into the Black men's market. The owners fired at the intruders, shooting one person. The Black men were arrested. Shortly after, deputies forcibly removed the men from jail and had them lynched, or hanged.

While many newspapers printed false information, Ida wrote about what actually happened. She told Black Americans not to shop at white-owned businesses, and they listened. White businessmen began to lose money. They broke into Ida's office and destroyed her printing presses. Fearing for her life, Ida fled to Chicago.

In Chicago, Ida continued writing about acts of racism in the United States. Her writing often focused on ending the practice of lynching. In 1892, she even published a pamphlet entitled *Southern Horrors: Lynch Law in All Its Phases*. In the pamphlet, she outlined the history of lynching and stated that it was a practice used to prevent Black people from moving forward in society. Ida even encouraged Black men to combat lynching with violence, a claim that was criticized by many.

Later, Ida helped found one of the most influential organizations for Black people that still exists today, the National Association for the Advancement of Colored People (NAACP). Since its founding in 1909, the NAACP has been a leader in securing justice for people of color. Ida did not remain active in the organization for long. She often argued with its leaders because she did not believe they were **militant** enough. While most leaders of the civil rights organization promoted racial equality by using **civil disobedience** to challenge unjust laws, Ida thought that racial inequality should be combated with force.

In the early 20th century, Black women were discouraged from participating in the civil rights movement because of their gender. They were also discouraged from participating in the women's suffrage movement because of their race. Women of color wanted to join the fight for equality, too, but it seemed no one would let them.

Ida addressed the treatment of Black Americans in the women's suffrage movement. Most suffrage groups did not want to involve people of color. They feared that would prevent them from winning the vote in the

South. White suffragists often laughed at Ida when she confronted them about this problem.

Since most large women's rights organizations would not allow women of color to join, Ida formed the Alpha Suffrage Club (ASC) to include Black Americans in the suffrage movement. The ASC not only worked to secure women's right to vote, but also to educate Black men and women about political leaders and processes. Ida believed that educating Black voters would ensure that more people were elected who supported causes important to women and all people of color.

In 1913, the first major parade of the women's suffrage movement was held in Washington, DC. Thousands of suffragists planned to march through the city while carrying signs that demanded the right to vote. When Ida and 60 other Black women arrived to march in the parade, they were told to stand in the back. Ida declared, "Either I go with you or not at all." Despite protests, she marched alongside the white suffragists. Pictures of Ida and the other Black women marching were published in newspapers throughout the country, bringing attention to the role of Black women in politics.

In her later years, Ida continued to write and fight for the rights of Black Americans. In 1930, she ran for a seat in Illinois's State Senate. Even though she lost, she was recognized as one of the first Black women to run for office. Ida died about a year later.

During her lifetime, Ida gave Black women a voice in the suffrage movement. By creating the ASC, she gave Black American women a place of **inclusion** in the movements that tried to leave them out. She also brought Black Americans' issues to the front pages of American journalism.

Her legacy continues to impact journalists today. In 1983, the first Ida B. Wells Award was given by the National Association of Black Journalists. Since then, the organization has continued to give the award to a journalist each year to recognize journalism that increases awareness about issues related to Black people.

EXPLORE MORE! Want to see the complete list of journalists who have received the Ida B. Wells Award and learn more about their work? Check out the National Association of Black Journalists website at NABJ.org.

DID YOU KNOW? During the early 20th century, there were about 200 lynchings per year in the United States. Most were of Black men living in the South. In Southern states, the threat of lynching was used to keep Black Americans from voting and to continue white supremacy.

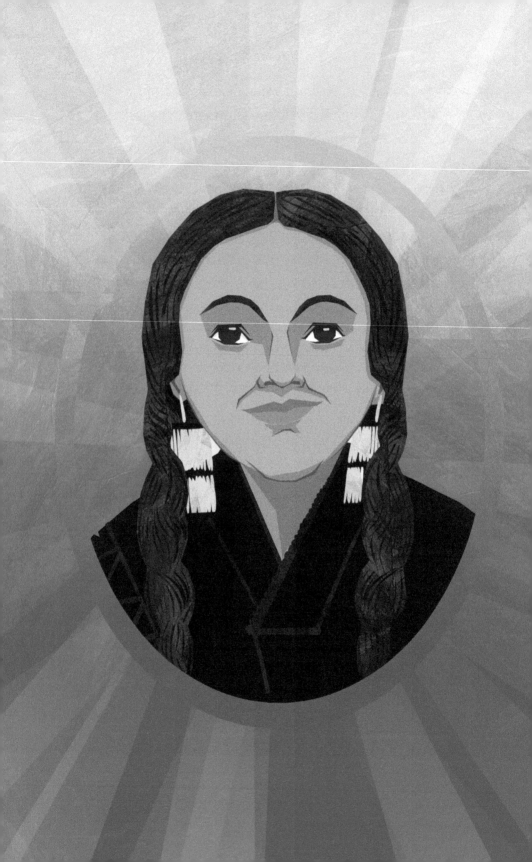

Marie Louise Bottineau
BALDWIN
1863–1952

What is something that makes you unique? Have you ever been afraid to share this with others because you were scared of what they may think or say? For many years, Marie Louise Bottineau Baldwin kept the thing that made her unique hidden. Eventually, she realized that prevented her from being her true self. By allowing her true self to show, Marie helped Indigenous people throughout the United States.

Marie was born into the Turtle Mountain Band of Chippewa Tribe in North Dakota. Her father was a lawyer who promoted the rights of the Chippewa and Ojibwa tribes. After finishing school, Marie went to work at her father's law office so that she could also help her people.

In the 1890s, Marie and her father moved to Washington, DC. While living in the Midwest, they were only able to help the tribes in that region. By moving to the nation's capital, they were able to help

Indigenous people throughout the country. Most of their work involved defending **treaty** rights for Indigenous people. Treaty rights had to do with the rights granted to tribes by the government, such as the right to occupy certain regions, hunting and fishing rights, and access to healthcare.

Marie's work fighting for the rights of Indigenous Americans did not go unnoticed. In 1904, President Theodore Roosevelt made Marie a clerk in the Office of Indian Affairs (OIA). (The words "Indian" and "Native American" were used before "Indigenous.") The purpose of the OIA was to build relationships and make treaties with Indigenous tribes.

Even though Marie was good at her job, she was not treated equally. She was paid $1,000 per year to work for the OIA. While this made her the highest-paid Indigenous woman at the office, her salary was still only about half of what others were paid. Most white clerks were paid $1,800 per year.

Early in her career, Marie believed that Indigenous people needed to become more like white Americans. She argued that it was best for them to dress like white people and try to fit in. After her father died in 1911, Marie's views changed. She no longer believed Indigenous tribes should give up their culture to fit into a society that stole tribal lands.

Shortly after her father's passing, Marie joined the Society of American Indians (SAI). The SAI was the first national Indigenous rights organization. Its members worked to preserve Indigenous culture and to advance issues important to Indigenous Americans. Marie became a leader within the organization and spoke at many of its meetings.

> **"IT IS NOT THE INDIAN WHO NEEDS TO BE EDUCATED SO CONSTANTLY UP TO THE WHITE MAN, BUT THAT THE WHITE MAN NEEDS TO BE EDUCATED TO THE INDIAN."**

The mission of the SAI strengthened Marie's new passion for maintaining Indigenous traditions. It was this passion that led Marie to do something considered **radical** at the time. All government workers were required to have official portraits taken. Marie posed for her portrait wearing traditional tribal clothing and two long braids. The photograph represented the importance of maintaining cultural traditions even when Indigenous peoples were expected to act like white Americans. After the photograph was taken, Marie began wearing the traditional clothing more frequently to public events.

In 1912, Marie followed in her father's footsteps by enrolling in law school. It takes most people three years to complete law school, but Marie earned her law degree in just two years, all while working a full-time job. She was also recognized as the first woman of color to graduate from the Washington College of Law.

Marie also became an active member of the women's suffrage movement when she realized the right to vote was a way to protect Indigenous culture. If Indigenous women could vote, they could vote for leaders and laws that protected the interests of their people. Marie met with Indigenous women throughout the United States, was interviewed by newspapers, and spoke in Congress about the importance of women's suffrage. Many recognized her as the voice for Indigenous women.

Just as the women's suffrage movement was not welcoming of Black women, the movement was also not welcoming of Indigenous women. In 1913, at the first major women's suffrage parade, Marie was told to march in the back of the parade with other women of color. Marie refused and marched alongside white female lawyers in the middle of the parade.

In 1914, President Woodrow Wilson invited a small group of women's suffrage leaders to meet with him at the White House. Marie was one of the only women of color invited to join the meeting. The women spoke to the president about the need for a women's suffrage amendment. The president declined to support the amendment at the time, but eventually spoke out in favor of women's suffrage.

Today, few people recognize the name Marie Louise Bottineau Baldwin. But her status as a hidden figure in

US history does not reduce her impact. Marie's work and willingness to openly display Indigenous culture led to greater equality for Indigenous people, especially Indigenous women. Recently, the Smithsonian acknowledged Marie's contributions by identifying her as one of the most important forgotten heroes of the suffrage movement on its website.

EXPLORE MORE! You can learn more about the history of Indigenous rights by taking a virtual field trip to the National Museum of the American Indian, at AmericanIndian.si.edu.

DID YOU KNOW? In 1851, Congress passed the Indian Appropriations Act, which forced Indigenous tribes to leave their homelands and settle on government-created reservations. The reservations stripped away Indigenous culture. Since they were not allowed to leave the reservations, many tribes also had to give up hunting and learn how to farm. The government encouraged those living on reservations to convert to Christianity and wear the same clothing worn by white Americans. Enemy tribes were also forced to live together on small plots of land, leading to conflicts.

Mary McLeod
BETHUNE
1875–1955

Have you ever experienced something so special that you wanted others to experience it, too? Mary McLeod Bethune was the first in her family to receive an education. Recognizing the opportunities that education brought her, she made it her life's mission to ensure others could receive an education, too.

Mary was born in South Carolina in 1875 to free parents who had been enslaved before the 13th Amendment abolished slavery. She was the first in her family to be born into freedom. Mary's parents worked for their former enslaver until they could afford to buy their own farm. Mary spent her early years working alongside her parents.

When Mary was 10 years old, she received funding to attend school. This was an opportunity few Black American children in the South were given. Mary wanted to learn to read and write so that she could become a **missionary** and teach people in Africa about

Christianity. After she graduated, Southern churches refused to send a Black missionary to Africa.

Since Mary was unable to go to Africa, she looked for ways to help Black Americans at home. She recognized that learning to read and write had changed her life and gave her new opportunities. Mary became an educator so that she could help Black children learn to read and write. She began by teaching at a school she had attended, but dreamed of opening her own school for Black girls.

"THE WHOLE WORLD OPENED TO ME WHEN I LEARNED TO READ AND WRITE."

In 1904, Mary's dream became a reality. She opened the Daytona Literary and Industrial Training School for Negro Girls in Florida. The school started with only five girls. When Mary was not teaching, she went door-to-door to raise money for the school. Eventually, it grew to include all grade levels and merged with an all-boys school. In 1931, the school became an accredited college, and its name changed to Bethune-Cookman University.

Of Mary's many accomplishments, Bethune-Cookman University was her biggest source of pride. She served as its first president until 1947. Even after she stepped down as president, she was involved with the school and its students. It was tough not to be involved, since she built her home on the campus.

Mary became active in the women's suffrage movement while growing her school. She was able to provide hundreds of Black children with an education, but there were still thousands throughout the South who were uneducated. Also, schools for Black children did not get the same resources and funding as white schools. If Black women were given voting rights, they would support laws to improve education for all Black children.

Mary joined several women's rights organizations and worked to educate other Black women on the importance of women's voting rights. But Mary's work to promote voting rights only began with the 19th Amendment.

Even after women received the right to vote, Southern laws made it almost impossible for Black women and men to vote. Mary was determined to find ways around those laws. When Black people were required to pay a fee to vote, she raised money to pay those fees. When white hate groups tried to scare Black Americans away from the polls, Mary led a parade of 100 Black Americans to the voting booths.

Mary also made sure Black women took advantage of their new political power. She formed the National Council of Negro Women (NCNW) to inspire Black women to participate in political activities and advocate for more opportunities for Black Americans. Mary served as the first president of the NCNW until 1949. During that time, the organization grew to more than 850,000 members.

Throughout the remainder of her life, Mary did everything she could to ensure that Black voices were heard. Her work to secure equality for all people was recognized at the highest levels of government. Mary served as an adviser to Presidents Calvin Coolidge and Herbert Hoover, encouraging them to create more opportunities for Black American children and youth.

Mary played an even bigger role in government during Franklin D. Roosevelt's presidency. President Roosevelt appointed Mary to be the leader of the National Youth Administration (NYA), making her the first Black American woman to lead a **federal agency**. The goal of the NYA was to create education and work opportunities for Americans between the ages of 16 and 25. Mary was also the only woman on President Roosevelt's Federal Council on Negro Affairs, which was also called the "Black Cabinet." The Black Cabinet advised the president on issues related to Black American rights.

Around 1949, Mary retired to her home on Bethune-Cookman University's campus, although her work was not done. She continued to **mentor** youth and host political leaders, sharing the importance of equality with all who entered her home. She also started a project to compile records that tell about the contributions Black American women have made to American history, known as the National Archives for Black Women's History.

Mary passed away in 1955, leaving behind many institutions that continue to impact American life. Today,

Bethune-Cookman University educates more than 2,900 students each year. The NCNW and its 2 million members continue to advocate for equality and opportunities for Black Americans. Finally, the National Archives for Black Women's History continues to serve as the only archive dedicated to the history of Black American women.

EXPLORE MORE! You can learn more about Mary's legacy by visiting Bethune-Cookman University in Daytona, Florida. In addition to touring the campus, you can visit her home and see a memorial in her honor.

DID YOU KNOW? After constitutional amendments gave all Americans the right to vote, laws were passed in Southern states to keep people of color from voting. Southern states required Black Americans to pay a poll tax and pass a literacy test to vote. These laws did not apply to white people. Most Black men and women in the South did not know how to read or write and, therefore, could not pass the literacy test. Of the ones that did pass the test, few could afford to pay the poll tax.

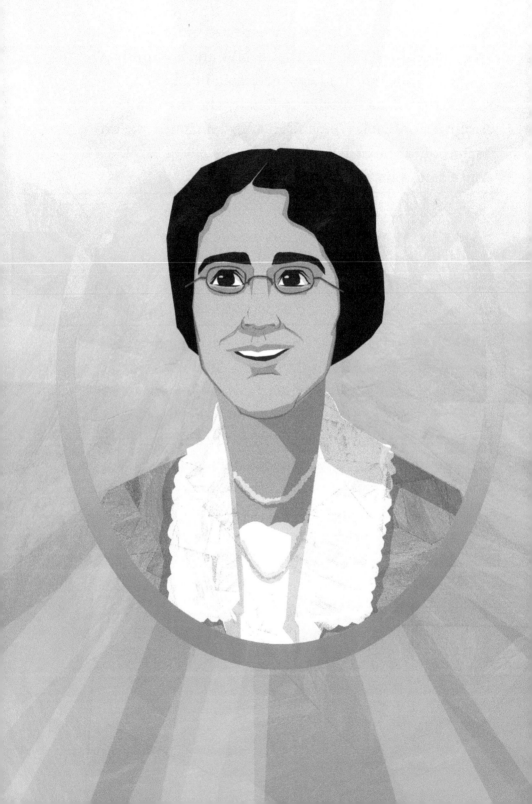

Adelina "Nina"
OTERO-WARREN
1881–1965

More than 11,500 constitutional amendments have been proposed in Congress since 1789, but only 27 have been added to the Constitution. That is because the process to **ratify** an amendment is lengthy. In addition to being approved by two-thirds of Congress, an amendment must also be approved by two-thirds of states. Getting two-thirds of states to agree on an amendment is no easy feat! The suffragists soon realized that to get Southwest states on board, they needed help from Spanish-speaking Americans. Adelina "Nina" Otero-Warren led the women's suffrage fight in New Mexico.

Nina was born in 1881 to a wealthy family in what is present-day New Mexico. The New Mexico Territory was a diverse region with Hispanic, Indigenous, and white American cultures present. Nina's father was killed when she was not even two years old, and her mother remarried a European man who was an **immigrant** to the United States. Nina's family wealth afforded her the opportunity to attend boarding school, where she received an advanced education that was not available to all women at the time.

After returning from school, Nina's family moved to Santa Fe. Her cousin was the governor of the New Mexico Territory and appointed her stepfather to a government position in the region. Having family at the highest levels of government led Nina to wealthy circles of people. She attended parties and mingled with political leaders. The political connections she made became important when Nina joined the women's suffrage movement a few years later.

In 1908, Nina married a military officer, Rawson Warren. The marriage ended two years later. In the early 20th century, divorced women were looked down upon. To avoid **prejudice**, Nina pretended to be widowed and kept her last name hyphenated.

Soon after her divorce, Nina became involved in the women's suffrage movement. She had grown up surrounded by political leaders, but had never been able to participate in government. Nina joined women's suffrage groups and spoke out in support of the movement.

While the women's suffrage movement did not always welcome people of color, suffrage leaders began to realize they had a problem. A women's suffrage amendment would need to be approved by at least 36 states to pass. The amendment would need the support of Spanish-speaking people to pass in states with large numbers of Hispanics, such as New Mexico.

The suffrage leader Alice Paul (page 51) heard about Nina's work in New Mexico and asked Nina to lead the New Mexico chapter of the Congressional Union for Woman Suffrage (CU). The CU was created to promote women's suffrage through petitions, speaking tours, parades, and meetings. It eventually became the National Woman's Party, the first political party created to promote women's rights.

> "[NINA] HAD READ ENOUGH HISTORY TO KNOW OTHERS FELT AS SHE DID ABOUT THE GRIEVOUS INEQUALITY OF WOMEN IN A NATION THAT PRIDED ITSELF ON GUARANTEEING FREEDOM AND JUSTICE FOR ALL."
> —CHARLOTTE WHALEY

Nina advocated for women's suffrage materials to be presented in both English and Spanish. She ensured that all pamphlets and reading materials were printed in both languages and that Spanish-speaking suffragists were present at events to give speeches.

Nina also used her political connections to push the women's suffrage amendment forward in New Mexico. Nina's persistence paid off. New Mexico ratified the 19th Amendment on February 21, 1920. A few months later, in August 1920, the 36th state ratified the amendment, adding it to the Constitution. Nina played a significant role in the amendment's ratification in New Mexico.

In 1922, Nina became the first Hispanic woman to run for US Congress when she campaigned to represent New Mexico in the US House of Representatives. She lost the election by only a few thousand votes, but continued to promote political causes that were important to her throughout the rest of her life.

Nina never had children, but she made helping the children in New Mexico a top priority. In 1917, she was made the leader of the public school system in Santa Fe, a position she held for more than 10 years. At the time, the government wanted Hispanics and Indigenous people to become more like white Americans. That meant giving up their language, traditional dress, and culture. Nina worked with the government to ensure that students in her schools could keep their cultural identities. She fought for English and Spanish to be allowed in the schools, even though there were laws that said only English could be spoken.

In the 1930s, Nina moved to a ranch outside of Santa Fe, where she lived a quiet life with her partner Mamie Meadors until she passed away in 1965. She spent time writing and building the ranch. Even though she was not active in politics during her later years, her early political work helped pave the way for the passage of the women's suffrage amendment and for New Mexicans maintaining their cultural identities.

EXPLORE MORE! Learn about Maria Guadalupe Evangelina de Lopez, another Latina who played an important role in the women's suffrage movement, by visiting WomensHistory.org. (Enter "Maria Guadalupe Evangelina de Lopez" in the search box.)

DID YOU KNOW? Turning a territory into a state is a long process. First, the people of the territory must vote to prove they favor statehood. If a majority of citizens vote to become a state, the territory can petition the US Congress. They must also create a territorial government and write a constitution that upholds the US constitution. Finally, the US Congress must vote in favor of statehood, and the president must sign a resolution recognizing the territory as a state. New Mexico completed this process and became a US state in 1912.

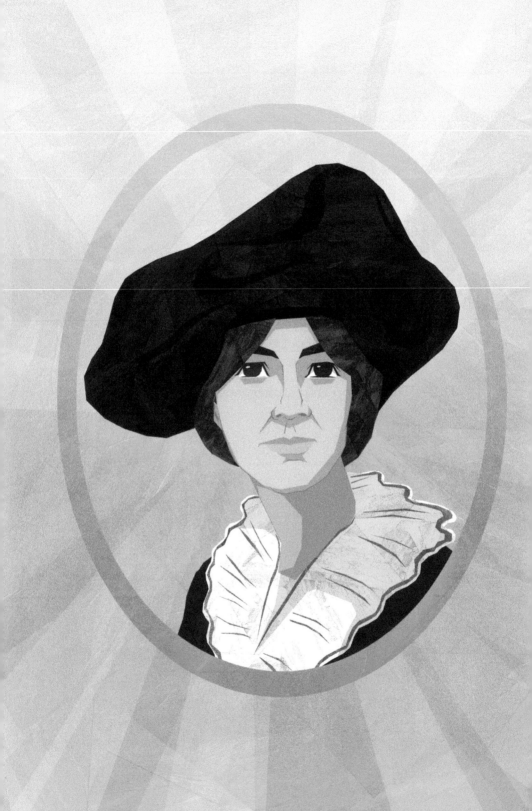

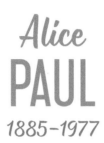

Alice
PAUL
1885–1977

Not all suffragists fought for the right to vote the same way. The early suffragists used writing and speeches to promote equality. Later, suffragists used more radical methods to get attention. Alice Paul was the first American suffrage activist to use militant protesting. This form of protest brought women's suffrage into the national spotlight.

Like other suffragists, such as Susan B. Anthony (page 9), Alice was raised by a Quaker family. The Quaker faith taught the importance of gender equality. Alice and her sisters were always treated the same as their brothers. Alice even attended women's suffrage meetings with her mother.

In the late 19th century, most women were expected to work in the home and raise their children. So, many did not believe that women needed an education. Alice's family thought differently. They believed in the importance of education, even for women. After earning several college degrees, Alice went to England to study. There, women were also fighting for the right to vote, but they used different methods. They led parades, picketed at government buildings, and broke windows. These actions made weekly headlines. Alice realized the US suffrage movement needed more public attention. She returned to the United States armed with new militant strategies.

> "MOST REFORMS, MOST PROBLEMS ARE COMPLICATED. BUT TO ME THERE IS NOTHING COMPLICATED ABOUT ORDINARY EQUALITY."

In 1913, Alice organized the suffrage movement's first major parade. More than 8,000 women carried signs from the US Capitol Building to the White House, demanding the right to vote. More than half a million people lined the streets to watch. Some gathered in support. But others were not as friendly. An angry mob of men yelled hateful words and even pushed the women. Some women were injured, but the police refused to stop the mob.

The violence brought national attention to the parade and women's suffrage. Many were upset to see women treated so poorly by their fellow Americans. Shortly after, President Woodrow Wilson agreed to meet with Alice and a few other suffragists. The president told the women he did not feel it was the right time for a suffrage amendment.

Alice was not only opposed by the president, but by other suffragists as well. Many women feared Alice's violent methods would anger government leaders and prevent women from getting the right to vote. They believed it was best to persuade leaders by writing, giving speeches, and trying to **lobby** Congress. Since most women's suffrage organizations would only let Alice join if she gave up her militant ways, Alice formed the Congressional Union for Woman Suffrage (CU). The CU led parades, held street meetings, collected signatures on petitions, hung billboards, and organized train tours of suffrage leaders.

In 1917, the National Woman's Party (NWP) was born from the CU. The NWP was the first political party designed to promote women's rights and equality. Like the CU, the NWP used militant strategies to raise awareness about issues related to women.

Today, it is not uncommon to see people protesting outside the White House. In 1917, Alice was the first to picket the White House. For 18 months, more than 1,000 members of the NWP took turns marching with signs outside the president's home. They were named the Silent Sentinels. At first, spectators ignored the women. After the United States entered World War I, the spectators turned violent. They believed protesting during wartime was unpatriotic. The women were called names, spit on, and pushed.

The police arrested Alice and other protestors for stopping traffic. Many thought the arrest was a violation of the First Amendment, which grants the freedom of speech. The women were put in cold, rat-infested prison cells for months. Many of the women were beaten by the prison guards. Alice led hunger strikes and refused to eat. Doctors threatened to send her to an insane asylum and force-fed her with tubes. Today, force-feeding is considered a form of torture.

Stories of the women in prison made headlines. The public was shocked by what they read. The NWP sent the women who had been jailed on speaking tours once they got out, and they talked about the harsh treatment they received. That helped build sympathy toward the suffragists. The public response forced President Wilson to change his position on women's suffrage. Soon after, the 19th Amendment was ratified.

Alice's work did not end with the 19th Amendment. Even though women were given the right to vote, they still were not treated as equals. Alice wrote the Equal Rights Amendment (ERA) in 1923. It read, "Men and women shall have equal rights throughout the United States and every place subject to its jurisdiction." Alice spent the rest of her life fighting to get it passed.

The ERA was brought to Congress every year between 1923 and 1972. It passed in 1972, but never received enough state votes to be added to the Constitution. Most amendments are given a seven-year time limit to be ratified. Congress extended the time line of the ERA to 1982, but it still did not receive enough state votes. As of 2021, the amendment is still being debated.

Alice passed away in 1977, but her legacy lives on through the NWP. The party has remained a voice for women in the United States. Since the 1920s, it has promoted equality for women in all aspects of life, including property rights, fair treatment in the workplace, and rights for divorced women. The party has also helped many women get elected to office and continues to seek equality for women under the Constitution by advocating for the passage of the ERA.

EXPLORE MORE! Learn more about the efforts of the National Woman's Party to pass the Equal Rights Amendment and how you can get involved by visiting NationalWomansParty.org.

DID YOU KNOW? Women in the United Kingdom were also fighting for the right to vote in the early 20th century. There, women who met certain requirements were allowed to vote in 1918. The British suffragists continued their fight until all women over the age of 21 could vote in 1928.

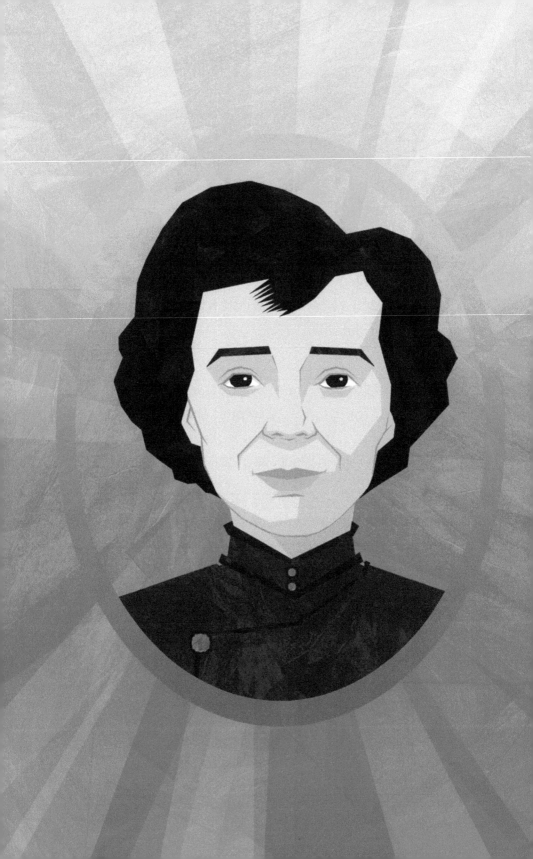

Mabel
PING-HUA LEE
1897–1966

Have you ever done something difficult just because it was the right thing to do? Not all women were able to vote, even after the 19th Amendment was ratified. Mabel Ping-Hua Lee knew a women's suffrage amendment would still not give her a voice in elections, but she chose to fight for the amendment anyway because helping other women gain political freedom was the right thing to do.

The United States passed the Chinese Exclusion Act in 1882. Chinese immigrants were willing to work for less money, which caused Americans to be overlooked for jobs. Many were unhappy that Chinese immigrants took jobs away from American citizens, so the government passed laws that made it tough for the Chinese to immigrate to the United States. The laws only allowed Chinese students, merchants, and missionaries to enter the country, but they were not allowed to bring their spouses and children with them.

Mabel was born in China in 1897. When she was four years old, her father moved to the United States to be a Christian missionary, or a person who spreads Christianity. American laws prevented her father from bringing her with him. So, Mabel stayed in China with her mother.

Mabel attended a school in China, where she learned to speak English. She excelled in her studies and was recognized for her work ethic. When she was nine years old, she received a scholarship that allowed her to move to the United States to attend school. In 1905, she moved to Chinatown in New York City with her father. Even though she attended school with students of different racial and cultural backgrounds, living in Chinatown allowed Mabel to remain close to her Chinese heritage.

By the time Mabel was 16 years old, she was considered a leader of the women's suffrage movement. She wrote essays for magazines and pamphlets, arguing that the United States would only have a successful democracy when women were given the right to vote. Many could not believe that someone so young could write such powerful arguments, and she caught the attention of the **media**. Articles about her work in the suffrage movement were published in some of the country's biggest newspapers.

The women's suffrage movement was not always accepting of women of color. But suffrage leaders felt they could learn from Chinese Americans. In the early 20th century, the Chinese Revolution took place in China, which led to increased rights for women. American suffragists looked to the events that had taken place in China for inspiration in their movement.

In 1912, Mabel led a major women's suffrage parade through New York City. She rode a horse as thousands of women marched behind her, waving signs. Thousands of people lined the streets to watch Mabel and her fellow suffragists march by. The parade brought attention to the women's suffrage movement, as it was photographed and covered in newspapers throughout the United States.

> **"[FEMINISM] IS NOTHING MORE THAN THE EXTENSION OF DEMOCRACY OR SOCIAL JUSTICE AND EQUALITY OF OPPORTUNITIES TO WOMEN."**

The Women's Political Union, a group that supported women's suffrage, opened a suffrage shop in 1915. The shop sold traditional goods while promoting the women's movement. For example, it sold soap wrapped in a pamphlet that described the reasons why women should be given the right to vote. The shop also hosted events and speakers to promote the cause.

Mabel was invited to be one of the first speakers at the Suffrage Shop. In a famous speech titled "The Submerged Half," Mabel encouraged members of the Chinese community to promote education and political equality for women. The speech was covered by the *New York Times* newspaper and received attention from both women's groups and the Chinese American community.

In 1917, New York gave women the right to vote. The 19th Amendment extended the right to all states in 1920, but many women were still banned from voting. The Chinese Exclusion Act prevented Chinese immigrants from becoming citizens. Without citizenship, Chinese Americans were unable to vote. Additional laws were passed throughout the early 20th century that placed even more restrictions on Chinese immigrants, leading many to question whether they would ever be able to participate in government. While Mabel had helped millions of women gain political freedom, she still had to fight for her own rights.

Mabel continued to write and speak about equality for women and Chinese Americans while attending college. At the time, few women pursued doctorate degrees. Mabel became the first Chinese woman to receive a doctorate degree in economics, giving her the title of Dr. Mabel Ping-Hua Lee.

After her father passed away, Mabel took over his position at the First Chinese Baptist Church of New York City. She worked as a pastor at the church and founded the Chinese Christian Center. The center provided job training, healthcare, English classes, and a kindergarten to Chinese immigrants. She used the center to continue advocating for the Chinese American community until she passed away in 1966.

Not much documentation was kept on Mabel's later years. The Chinese Exclusion Act ended in 1943, allowing Chinese Americans to become US citizens. No one knows whether Mabel ever pursued citizenship or voted, but her work in the suffrage movement had a lasting impact on all women, especially Chinese Americans. In 2018, New York City's Chinatown post office was named after her to honor her work for the community.

EXPLORE MORE! Learn about other women of color who have been left out of the history of the women's suffrage movement by visiting AmericanHistory.si.edu /creating-icons/who-was-left-out-story.

DID YOU KNOW? Many Chinese immigrants came to the United States during the mid-1800s. Most chose to live and work close together because of racial prejudices and **hate crimes** directed at Chinese immigrants. Many Chinese immigrants settled in lower Manhattan, and the area became known as Chinatown. The community was known for maintaining Chinese traditions through food and celebrations.

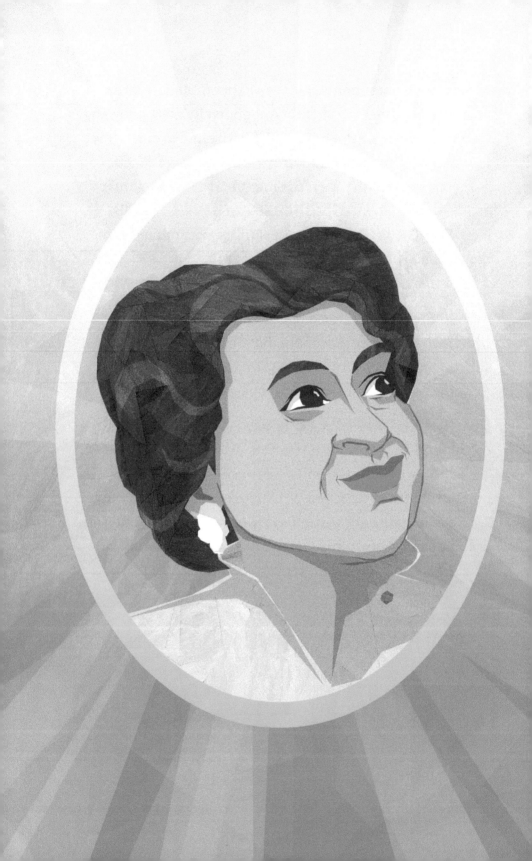

Betty
FRIEDAN
1921–2006

During the mid-20th century, magazines featured American women wearing dresses and pearl necklaces as they cleaned and cooked. The women were always smiling and happy, which led society to believe that this is how all women should act. Betty Friedan started the modern feminist movement after writing a book that exposed the reality of being an American housewife.

Betty was born to immigrant parents in 1921. With her mother's encouragement, Betty earned a college degree. She even trained to be a psychologist for a short time, before dropping out of school to join the workforce. As a student, Betty was involved in supporting several political causes. She wrote pamphlets that encouraged workplace equality, especially for women.

During World War II, Betty worked as a reporter. Even though she was a skilled writer, she was forced to give up her job to a man who returned from the war. After the war, Betty took a job as a psychologist, but was fired again for taking maternity leave after giving birth to her second child. She began working from home as a freelance writer for women's magazines.

At a college reunion, Betty surveyed her classmates. She found that nearly 90 percent were not using their education in their roles as housewives. Most of the women were not happy in their roles inside the home. This revelation led Betty on a five-year journey to learn more about gender roles, or what is expected from men and women. She interviewed women across the country who felt trapped in their gender roles. Women wanted to find satisfaction outside of the home but lacked opportunities.

"A GIRL SHOULD NOT EXPECT SPECIAL PRIVILEGES BECAUSE OF HER SEX, BUT NEITHER SHOULD SHE 'ADJUST' TO PREJUDICE AND DISCRIMINATION."

Betty tried to publish her findings in magazines. No magazine would work with her, so she turned the information into a book. In 1963, a publisher agreed to publish *The Feminine Mystique*. The book was an instant bestseller. Betty's writing made women question their roles in society and led to the start of the modern feminist movement, which is also known as the women's liberation movement. Today, *The Feminine Mystique* is considered one of the most influential books of the 20th century.

The Feminine Mystique identified what Betty referred to as "the problem that has no name" in speaking about women's discontent with their gender roles. After her book's success, Betty wanted to find ways to solve that unnamed problem. She cofounded the National Organization for Women (NOW) to advocate for women's issues and promote gender equality in all areas of life. Betty served as the president for several years. In that role, she was successful in ending gender-specific job listings.

In 1970, on the 50th anniversary of the women's suffrage amendment, Betty and NOW organized the Women's Strike for Equality. Women stopped working for one day to raise awareness about unequal pay. Tens of thousands of women skipped work. Instead, they marched and protested in cities throughout the United States. The nation was listening. The next year, Congress declared the day "Women's Equality Day," even though women have yet to receive equal pay in the workplace.

After the strike, Betty cofounded the National Women's Political Caucus (NWPC) with other feminists, including Gloria Steinem (page 75). The goal of the organization is to achieve gender equality through political participation. Since its founding, the NWPC has played a leading role in promoting the Equal Rights Amendment. The NWPC has also been key in getting Congress to pass workplace equality laws. Thanks to the NWPC, laws have been passed that increased pay for women, ended unfair hiring practices, and prevented employers from not hiring women due to pregnancy.

Shortly after its founding, the NWPC launched the Win with Women campaign. The campaign increased the number of women elected to office through training and support. The organization offered training to help women understand how to run for office. It provided public support for any women who chose to pursue political office. When the NWPC was founded in 1971, only 15 women served in the US Congress. In 2020, 126 women held seats in Congress. Many credit the NWPC for this increase.

Though she has been called the "mother of the modern women's movement," Betty was criticized by other feminists for advocating only for white middle- and upper-class women. Betty's work gave a voice to many, but lower-class, gay women, and women of color were left out. Betty's opponents argued that her attitude toward women who were different from her threatened to destroy the women's movement.

Betty continued to promote women's rights legisla-tion, write books, and teach at a college until she died in 2006. Today, *The Feminine Mystique* is required reading in women's history classes. The book continues to reso-nate with women and impact the way gender roles are viewed. Since its release, millions of copies have been sold worldwide, and it has been translated into more than 10 languages. Many of the advancements women have made in the workplace are thanks to organizations founded by Betty, including NOW and the NWPC.

EXPLORE MORE! As one of the most influential books of the 20th century, a copy of *The Feminine Mystique* is included as an artifact at the Smithsonian's National Museum of American History. Take a virtual field trip to the Smithsonian by visiting SI.edu to examine the copy on display, and other artifacts related to the women's rights movements.

DID YOU KNOW? The modern feminist movement is still going on today. Women continue to fight for issues such as equal pay and stricter laws against harassment. Like the early suffragists, women continue to fight for their rights with marches and protests.

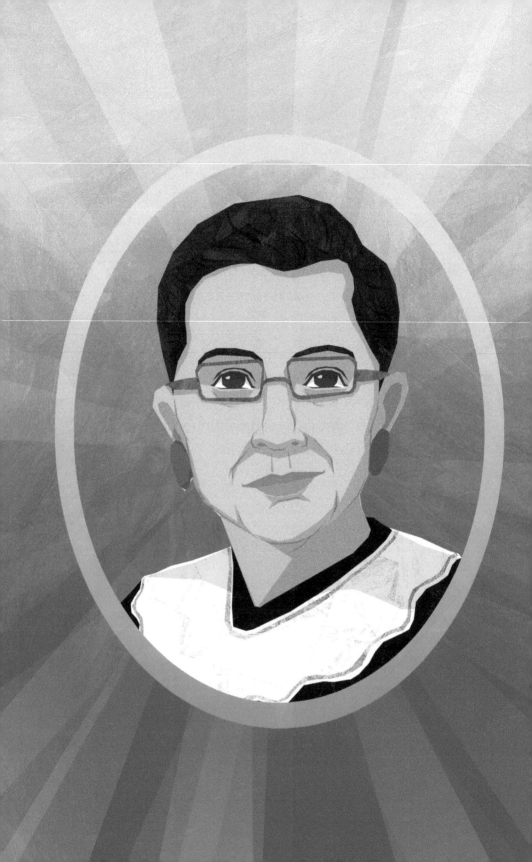

Ruth Bader
GINSBURG
1933–2020

Throughout the history of women's rights, women have sought greater equality by writing essays, giving speeches, hosting parades and events, and signing petitions. But Ruth Bader Ginsburg pursued gender equality differently. She earned a law degree and fought to change laws that discriminated against women.

Ruth was born in 1933 into a Jewish family living in New York. Her mother believed in the importance of education for girls. She encouraged Ruth to learn as much as possible and instilled in her a love for discovering new things.

In 1954, Ruth graduated at the top of her class from Cornell University. After graduating, she married Martin Ginsburg and they had two children. At the time, it was rare for women to pursue multiple college degrees, especially if they were married. Women were expected to stay home and take care of their children, but Ruth chose a different path. She decided to attend law school while raising her children.

Ruth was accepted into Harvard Law School, which is one of the oldest and best law schools in the United States. Of the 500 law students in her class, only 10 were women. She was often discriminated against by the male students and professors. Ruth was regularly accused by her professors of taking a seat away from a man. They said she should not have accepted a spot at the school so that a man could have the spot. The women were also not allowed to use certain sections of the library or read certain law books.

Through it all, Ruth let her work and grades do the talking. During her final year of law school, she transferred to Columbia University after her husband took a job in New York. Ruth graduated at the top of her class.

Ruth had trouble finding work after graduating. It was hard for women to find legal jobs due to discrimination, and it was even tougher for Jewish women. Ruth eventually took a job as a law clerk in a New York district court, where she worked for two years. After leaving that job, she worked at several law schools, researching court cases and teaching classes.

Ruth was most passionate about using the legal system to create gender equality. In 1971, she got the opportunity to play a leading role in the feminist movement. The American Civil Liberties Union (ACLU) is an organization that defends individual freedoms guaranteed under the Constitution. With the rise in the modern feminist movement in the 1960s, the ACLU formed a new division called the Women's Rights Project to help end discrimination against women. Ruth was asked to lead it.

As the leader of the Women's Rights Project, Ruth provided legal representation in court cases that involved discrimination toward women. Six of the cases she represented were held before the Supreme Court. She won five of those cases. Through her work with the ACLU, Ruth achieved greater equality for women in education, the workforce, and the military.

"WOMEN BELONG IN ALL PLACES WHERE DECISIONS ARE BEING MADE."

In 1980, President Jimmy Carter appointed Ruth to the US Court of Appeals for the District of Columbia. In the United States, cases are reviewed at different levels before they are sent to the US Supreme Court, which is the highest-ranking court. First, cases go before local and district courts. Then they are sent to a Court of Appeals, which provides the final review before the Supreme Court. Ruth worked for the Court of Appeals until 1993, when she was nominated by President Bill Clinton to serve as a Supreme Court justice.

As a justice, Ruth continued to support laws that favored gender equality and women's rights. One of her most important cases was *United States v. Virginia*. A woman had sued the Virginia Military Institute because the college refused to accept women. In the Supreme Court ruling, Ruth noted that government-funded schools could not deny admission to a man or woman if they were qualified to attend. The outcome of the case changed the US education system forever and provided more educational opportunities for women.

In another case, *Ledbetter v. Goodyear Tire & Rubber Co.*, a woman sued her employer after discovering that men in the same position were paid more. The Supreme Court ruled against the woman. This meant companies could continue paying male employees more. In her **dissent**, Ruth accused the male justices of being indifferent to gender equality in the workplace.

Ruth's outspokenness and unwavering dedication to equality earned her a famous nickname: the Notorious RBG. A college student gave Ruth the nickname, modeled after a rapper's name. The nickname stuck and came to symbolize her firmness and popularity.

Ruth remained a Supreme Court justice until she passed away in 2020. In her later years, she battled cancer, but it never stopped her from continuing her fight for justice. She was known to review and research cases from her hospital bed.

Few people have had as big of an impact on the modern feminist movement as Ruth. She overturned laws and practices that discriminated against women, paving the way for greater equality in the workplace, education, and everyday life.

EXPLORE MORE! Learn more about some of the most important cases in the history of the Supreme Court at USCourts.gov/about-federal-courts/educational -resources/supreme-court-landmarks.

DID YOU KNOW? In the history of the US Supreme Court, fewer than 5 percent of the justices have been women. As of 2021, there have been five female justices. Sandra Day O'Connor, Sonia Sotomayor, Elena Kagan, and Amy Coney Barrett also have served as Supreme Court justices. A woman has never been the leader of the Supreme Court, a position also known as the chief justice.

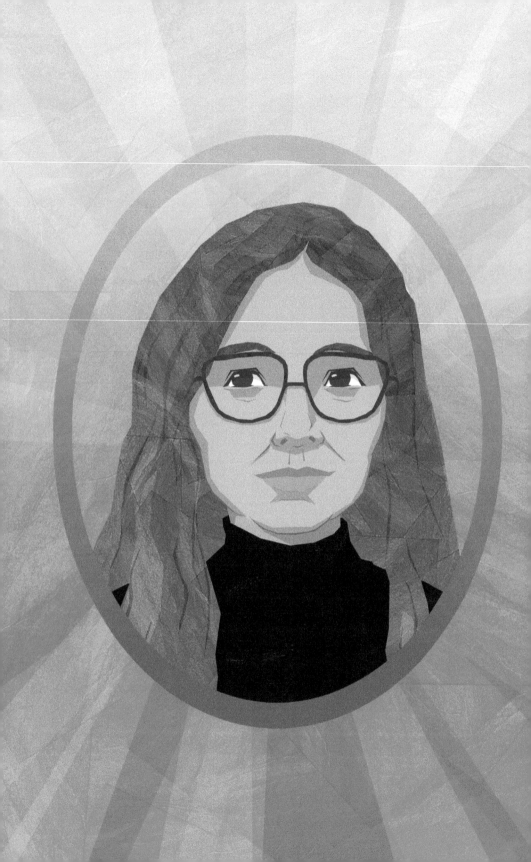

Gloria
STEINEM
1934–Present

Have you ever attended Take Our Daughters to Work Day? Each year, millions of young girls join the workplace for a day to learn about different careers. If you've ever participated in the event, you have Gloria Steinem to thank.

Gloria was born in Ohio in 1934. Her parents divorced when she was just 10 years old. Gloria had to take care of her mentally ill mother. These early experiences began to shape Gloria's feminist views, especially about marriage. In the 1950s, women were expected to take care of their husbands. After taking care of her mother for many years, Gloria declared that she was not interested in taking care of anyone ever again, and vowed to never marry. Although she did eventually marry in 2000, at the age of 66, the marriage did not last long, as her husband died a few years later.

After Gloria graduated from high school, her sister took over the care of their mother so that Gloria could attend college. She graduated with a degree in government. Soon after, Gloria received a scholarship to spend two years studying in India. It was in India that her political career truly began. She was inspired by the grassroots movements taking place. A grassroots movement is one where ordinary citizens from communities across the country work together to bring about change. This is different from a movement started by the government. The grassroots idea of leading from the bottom up rather than the top down is something Gloria later applied to the feminist movement.

> **"THE FIRST PROBLEM FOR ALL OF US, MEN AND WOMEN, IS NOT TO LEARN, BUT TO UNLEARN."**

Upon returning to the United States, Gloria worked as a journalist. She wanted to write about political issues, but was forced to write for the women's pages of newspapers and magazines. In the 1950s, "women's pages" contained information about fashion and housekeeping, but not about politics or current events. When she asked to write about politics, Gloria was told that she was not the right person to write about those topics.

Gloria decided that if the major newspapers and magazines would not take her seriously, she would start her own publication. In 1968, she cofounded *New York* magazine. The purpose of the magazine was to publish stories about New York politics and culture in a way that was more honest than most major publications. As editor, Gloria wrote a political column for the magazine, covering many important political and social issues, including the feminist movement.

Gloria's involvement in the feminist movement began around 1968. Before the 1973 *Roe v. Wade* Supreme Court decision that legalized abortions, each state had its own laws regarding abortions. In 1969, New York's state government held hearings to reform abortion laws. Feminists were outraged that the people selected to speak at the hearings were almost all men. A feminist group held a speak-out event to spread awareness about the women's rights issue.

Hundreds of people attended the event, where they heard women share their opinions about abortion. Gloria was one of the speakers. She shared a personal story about an abortion she had when she was younger. Her testimony was shocking, as it was not the norm for women to speak publicly about illegal abortions. After the event, Gloria was asked to speak at more women's rights events and protests. She quickly rose to become a leader within the movement.

As Gloria became more involved in the feminist movement, she was disappointed to see so few publications with articles about women's rights. Most women's magazines continued to only publish stories about fashion and housekeeping. In 1971, Gloria cofounded *Ms.* magazine to cover issues related to women's rights, such as workplace equality and domestic violence. The publication first appeared as an insert in *New York* magazine but became an independent magazine in 1972. Gloria worked as the editor of the magazine for 15 years. Today, she continues to select and write stories for the magazine.

Throughout the late 20th century, Gloria cofounded many organizations to promote gender equality and women's rights. In 1971, she cofounded the National Women's Political Caucus (NWPC) with other feminists, such as Betty Friedan (page 63). Over the past five decades, the NWPC has played an active role in helping more women get elected to public office.

With a background in journalism, Gloria remains passionate about how women are portrayed in the media. In 1971, she helped found the Women's Action Alliance (WAA). The WAA brought grassroots women's rights groups together through different projects. One of their projects involved creating children's books that support gender equality. In 2004, Gloria also founded the Women's Media Center to promote positive, powerful images of women in the media.

In 1986, Gloria was diagnosed with breast cancer, but she did not let the disease stop her work. She continues to play a role in women's movements. Since the 1980s, she has written several books and also cofounded countless organizations that promote women's rights throughout the world. In 1992, she also started Take Our Daughters to Work Day to expose young girls to the workplace. Today, millions of children participate in the event every April.

In 2013, Gloria received the highest nonmilitary award any US civilian can receive. President Barack Obama awarded Gloria the Presidential Medal of Freedom to honor her work and legacy for women's rights. Gloria has also been named one of the top 25 most influential American women by *Biography* and other magazines and has received many awards for her journalistic work. Gloria continues to fight for women's rights.

EXPLORE MORE! Want to learn more about Gloria? Read *Who Is Gloria Steinem?* by Sarah Fabiny.

DID YOU KNOW? Take Our Daughters to Work Day is no longer just for girls. In 2003, the program was expanded to include boys. Leaders of the program realized that true gender equality meant exposing both girls and boys to the workplace. Now it is referred to as either Take Our Children to Work Day or Take Our Daughters and Sons to Work Day.

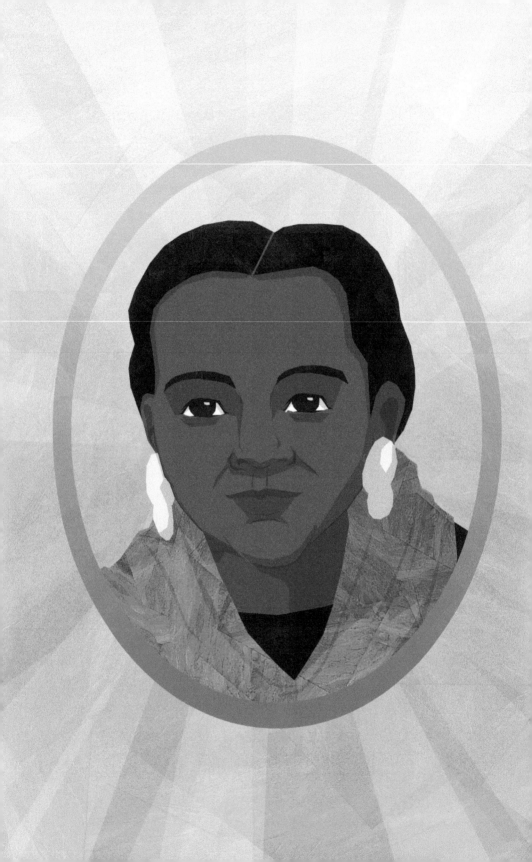

bell
hooks
1952–Present

A name can tell you a lot about a person. It may give you clues about family history or heritage. It can also hint at the spiritual or religious beliefs of a parent. What does your name say about you? To bell hooks, her name symbolized the voices of previous generations of women.

Gloria Watkins was born in Kentucky in 1952. Even though slavery had ended more than 80 years before she was born, the South did not treat Black people as equals. Some laws prevented them from having the same rights as white people. People of color were often separated from white people. Gloria lived in a **segregated** neighborhood and attended segregated schools. To escape the racial hatred of the time, she read poetry and wrote. By the time she was 10, Gloria started writing poetry and reciting it in church.

Gloria's family did not support her writing or encourage her to go to college. They believed that men should be the leader of their families, while the woman's role was to be a wife and mother. They also preached that women should follow their husbands' lead and do as they were told. Gloria opposed this view of family life. She rebelled against her family and went to college.

Gloria began writing her first book at the age of 19 while she was still in college. It was then that she decided to create a new identity. Initially, Gloria was afraid to share her ideas about gender and racial equality. Throughout her childhood, she had been afraid to express herself because of white hate groups in the South and her father's controlling influence. By creating a new identity, she felt empowered to write and speak about her beliefs.

Gloria changed her name to bell hooks, which was her great-grandmother's name. Traditionally, a father's last name is given to his wife and children. bell wanted to show that women leave legacies, too, by adopting her great-grandmother's name. She believed the name symbolized her female ancestors and their need to speak for themselves. She chose to write her name using all lowercase letters so that the focus would be on her message instead of herself.

Over eight years, bell took her first book to several publishers, but none would publish it. In 1981, after bell spoke at a feminist event, a publisher finally agreed to publish *Ain't I a Woman: Black Women and Feminism*. The book was inspired by Sojourner Truth's (page 15) speech by the same name. By describing the role of Black women throughout American history, it brought Black American women's concerns to the center of the feminist movement.

In the 1960s and '70s, the feminist movement mostly included white middle- and upper-class women. Even though the movement advocated for equality, women of color and poor women were left out. bell unveiled the racism taking place within the modern feminist movement and gave Black feminists a voice for the first time.

> ## "WHAT WE DO IS MORE IMPORTANT THAN WHAT WE SAY OR WHAT WE SAY WE BELIEVE."

Throughout her career, bell used her writing to reveal the multiple forms of discrimination that Black American women experience. They face gender discrimination for being female. They also face racial discrimination for being Black. bell noted that it is difficult for Black American women to find their places in society, since they face discrimination from more than one group and for more than one reason. She argued for gender and racial equality in all of her writings and speeches. This message of both gender and racial equality became known as "intersectional feminism."

The purpose of the modern feminist movement is that women gain social equality with men in all aspects of life. In her 1984 book, *Feminist Theory: From Margin to Center,* bell argued that the purpose of the movement should change. She presented the idea that the goal should be for people to recognize one another's differences and still accept everyone.

One of the reasons why people have responded to bell's writing is because she writes for everyone, not just the educated and the upper class. Even though her writing often presents big ideas about feminism, race, and class, she writes those ideas in a way that is easy to understand. bell believed that for people to engage in a movement, they have to be able to understand what the movement is about. Her easy-to-read style made her books popular with people from different backgrounds and led many to support the Black feminist movement.

Bell has written more than 30 books throughout her career as an activist and Black feminist. Her books include personal memoirs, poetry, and philosophies and theories about feminism. Since the 1980s, bell has also worked as a college professor. She has taught English, women's studies, and Black American studies at some of the best schools in the United States, including Yale University. In this role, she shares the message of equality with future generations.

In 2014, bell founded the bell hooks Institute at Berea College, where she has been teaching since 2004. The institute continues bell's research about the relation-ship between gender, race, and class to end systems of **oppression**. The institute also celebrates her work with a museum of artifacts in Kentucky that is open to the public. Thousands have learned about intersectional feminism by seeing the writings and artifacts on display at the institute.

~~~~~~

EXPLORE MORE! bell hooks has not only written books for adults. She has also written many children's books, including *Skin Again*, *Happy to Be Nappy*, and *Grump Groan Growl*. You can find bell's books wherever books are sold.

DID YOU KNOW? Because Black women were discriminated against for their gender and race, many did not believe they had a place in the feminist movement or the civil rights movement. In 1973, the National Black Feminist Organization (NBFO) was founded. The NBFO was one of few organizations to fight for both gender and racial equality.

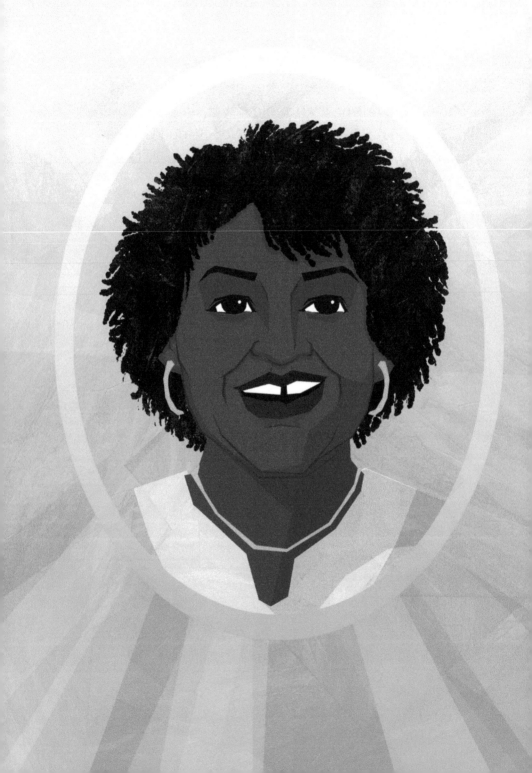

Stacey
ABRAMS
1973–Present

Even though the Constitution grants all Americans the right to vote regardless of color or gender, the fight for voter equality still has not ended. Voting rights is one of the most important and controversial topics in the United States today. Stacey Abrams continues the work of the suffragists who came before her by fighting for all Americans to have fair and equal access to the polls.

Stacey was born in Wisconsin in 1973. Her parents were ministers who encouraged their church to take care of the less fortunate. Throughout Stacey's childhood, her parents taught their children three core values: go to school, go to church, and take care of one another.

Stacey clung to those values while growing up, especially the part about going to school. She was her high school's first Black valedictorian. A valedictorian is the person who graduates with the best grades out of everyone in the class. After high school, Stacey went on to earn several college degrees, including a law degree from Yale University.

Stacey began her political career when she was just 17 years old, working as a speechwriter for a congressman's election campaign. She also held voter registration drives even though she was not yet old enough to vote. From an early age, Stacey saw the importance of empowering individuals to express their voices by voting and wanted all people to take advantage of this right.

> "EFFECTIVE LEADERS MUST BE TRUTH SEEKERS, AND THAT REQUIRES A WILLINGNESS TO UNDERSTAND TRUTHS OTHER THAN OUR OWN."

After law school, Stacey worked as a lawyer in Georgia. In 2006, Stacey was elected to the Georgia House of Representatives. Within a few years, she became the leader of the Democratic political party in the House, making her the first Black American to lead in the state's House of Representatives. While working as a lawyer and state representative, Stacey always advocated for poor and underserved communities.

After leaving Congress in 2017, Stacey ran for governor of Georgia, becoming the first Black woman in the United States to earn the nomination of a major political party when running for governor. On Election Day, she received more votes than any other Democratic candidate running for any office in the state's history. Despite her popularity, she lost the election by less than two percent of the votes.

Since the 19th century, there have been people in power who have tried to undo the 15th and 19th Amendments, which gave all Americans the right to vote. The South created poll taxes and literacy tests to keep people of color and the poor from voting. Later, laws were passed to keep certain immigrants from becoming citizens, thereby prohibiting them from voting. While most Americans might have assumed that no one was kept from voting in the 21st century, Stacey's governor election results proved that problems still exist.

Stacey's opponent worked for a government office that oversaw elections and voter registration. After the election, it was discovered that his office had canceled more than one million voter registrations without notifying most of the voters of the cancellation. The majority of those voters were people of color. The office also closed more than 200 polling places in poor neighborhoods, making it significantly more difficult for many to get out and vote.

These discoveries proved that the election was unfair. Thousands of people had been deliberately prevented from voting. After the election, Stacey chose to peacefully step down, but she refused to concede or admit defeat. In a speech, she stated, "Concession means to acknowledge an action is right, true, or proper. As a woman of conscience and faith, I cannot concede."

The outcome of the election made Stacey realize that the work of the early suffragists was not yet complete. The fight to ensure all people have fair and equal access to voting was only beginning. In 2018, Stacey founded the organization Fair Fight. The purpose of the organization is to encourage voter participation and educate voters about their voting rights. Fair Fight is credited with registering 800,000 new voters in Georgia before the 2020 presidential election. Most of the new voters were people of color and poor citizens.

Stacey also works to ensure that all American voices are heard through the US Census. Every 10 years, the government takes a census to count how many people are living in communities across the country. Often, people of color and poor Americans are left out of the census, so their communities do not receive as much funding or representation in government. In 2018, Stacey founded Fair Count. The organization aided in the 2020 Census to ensure fair and accurate counting took place in Georgia. Accurate counting meant funds and representation were distributed evenly across the state.

Today, Stacey continues to amplify the voices of Americans who are often left out of the political process. While Stacey's Fair Fight and Fair Count organizations have mostly helped the people of Georgia, Stacey hopes to expand these organizations throughout the country to ensure that all people have fair representation and the opportunity to express their most basic civic right, which is granted to all through the Constitution. Like the suffragettes and other female leaders who came before her, Stacey believes that every American deserves to have a voice in government.

EXPLORE MORE! Like Stacey, you're never too young to get involved in government. Learn more about Fair Fight and how you can play a role by visiting FairFight.com.

DID YOU KNOW? The practice of canceling voter registrations is required by law. Each state is expected to perform routine voter list maintenance, which involves canceling voter registrations for people who have died or moved to other states. In some states, voter registrations are also canceled if a person has not voted within a certain number of years. The practice is meant to help states save money, but it is sometimes taken advantage of to sway election results by inaccurately or unfairly canceling some registrations.

Glossary

abolitionist: A person who wants to end slavery

activist/activism: A person who actively works to bring about changes to the law or society; the act of doing so

citizen: A person who legally lives in a country and has the rights and protection of that country

civil disobedience: Protesting unfair laws peacefully

civil rights: The rights that every person should have regardless of race, gender, religion, etc.

discrimination: When a person or group is treated unfairly compared to others in society

dissent: An opinion written by a Supreme Court justice who disagrees with the majority opinion

equality: Having the same rights and opportunities

federal agency: A government organization that has a specific purpose, such as managing resources, overseeing financial institutions, or guarding national security

feminist: A person who believes in equal rights for women

hate crimes: Crimes or violent offenses against a person or group of people that is committed based on their race, gender, religion, sexuality, age, size, or ability

immigrant: A person who has moved to another country

inclusion: The act of including someone or something as part of a group

lobby: An attempt to persuade government leaders to support a specific cause

media: A form of communication designed to reach a large number of people, such as newspapers, magazines, television, social media, etc.

mentor: A person who teaches or advises a less-experienced or younger person

militant: Using extreme and sometimes violent methods to achieve something

missionary: A person sent to a foreign place to do religious work

movement: When a group of people work together to share a message or achieve a shared goal

oppression: To treat a person or group of people cruelly or unfairly, often for a long period of time

prejudice: Disliking a person or group of people because of their race, gender, religion, etc.

racism: Prejudice and discrimination toward a person or people because of their membership in a particular racial or ethnic group

radical: Very different or extreme; not ordinary

ratify: To give official approval

segregated: When one group of people is separated from another, often due to race, gender, wealth, or religion

treaty: An official agreement made by two or more groups

References

Alexander, Kerri Lee. "Frances Ellen Watkins Harper." National Women's History Museum, 2020. WomensHistory.org/education-resources/biographies /frances-ellen-watkins-harper.

Alexander, Kerri Lee. "Mabel Ping-Hua Lee." National Women's History Museum, 2020. WomensHistory.org /education-resources/biographies/mabel-ping-hua-lee.

Alexander, Kerri Lee. "Ruth Bader Ginsburg." National Women's History Museum, 2020. WomensHistory.org /education-resources/biographies/ ruth-bader-ginsburg.

Alice Paul Institute. "Equal Rights Amendment." Accessed March 30, 2021. EqualRightsAmendment.org.

Alice Paul Institute. "Who Was Alice Paul?" Accessed February 17, 2021. AlicePaul.org/about-alice-paul.

American Civil Liberties Union. "About the ACLU Women's Rights Project." Accessed February 23, 2021. ACLU.org/other/about-aclu-womens-rights-project.

Baker, Lee D. "Ida B. Wells-Barnett and Her Passion for Justice." Duke University. April 1996. People.Duke.edu /~ldbaker/classes/aaih/caaih/ibwells/ibwbkgrd.html.

Barrett, Whitney. "Mary McLeod Bethune: Educator & Activist." Historical Society of Central Florida. March 6, 2019. TheHistoryCenter.org/mcleod-bethune.

Brandman, Mariana. "Adelina Otero-Warren." National Women's History Museum, 2020. WomensHistory.org /education-resources/biographies/adelina-otero -warren.

Duignan, Brian, ed. "Elizabeth Cady Stanton." Encyclopedia Britannica, Inc., 2021. Britannica.com/biography /Elizabeth-Cady-Stanton.

Ehrlich, Jamie. "Ruth Bader Ginsburg's Most Notable Supreme Court Decisions and Dissents." Cable News Network. September, 18, 2020. CNN.com/2020/09/18/ politics/rbg-supreme-court-decisions-dissents/index. html.

Fair Fight. "About Stacey Abrams." Accessed February 26, 2021. FairFight.com/about-stacey-abrams.

Feigen, Brenda. "The ACLU, Ruth Bader Ginsburg, and Me." American Civil Liberties Union. May 27, 2020. ACLU.org/issues/womens-rights/aclu-ruth-bader -ginsburg-and-me.

Gender on the Ballot Team. "The National Women's Political Caucus: A Brief History." Gender on the Ballot. July 11, 2019. GenderOnTheBallot.org/nwpc.

Goodman, Elyssa. "How bell hooks Paved the Way for Intersectional Feminism." *Them.* March 12, 2019. them.us /story/bell-hooks.

Groer, Annie. "In India, Gloria Steinem Returns to the Roots of Her Activism." *The Washington Post*, January 20, 2014. WashingtonPost.com/lifestyle /style/in-india -steinem-returns-to-the-roots-of-her-activism/2014 /0½0/b6150c58-81f0-11e3-9dd4-e7278db80d86 _story.html.

Halsall, Paul. "Sojourner Truth: Ain't I a Woman?" National Park Service. Last modified January 20, 2021. NPS.gov/articles/sojourner-truth.htm.

Hayward, Nancy. "Susan B. Anthony." National Women's History Museum, 2018. WomensHistory.org/education -resources/biographies/susan-b-anthony.

History.com editors. "Ruth Bader Ginsburg." History, 2021. History.com/topics/womens-history/ruth-bader -ginsburg.

Igielnik, Ruth. "Men and Women in the U.S. Continue to Differ in Voter Turnout Rate, Party Identification." Pew Research Center. August 18, 2020. PewResearch.org /fact-tank/2020/08/18/men-and-women-in-the -u-s-continue-to-differ-in-voter-turnout-rate-party -identification.

Iowa State University. "Frances Ellen Watkins Harper." Accessed February 18, 2021. AWPC.cattcenter.iastate .edu/directory/frances-ellen-watkins-harper.

Janigro, Alice. "Ida B. Wells." Women's Suffrage Celebration Coalition. Accessed February 13, 2021. Suffrage100MA.org/ida-b-wells.

Jankowski, Lauren. "Biography of bell hooks, Feminist and Anti-Racist Theorist and Writer." Thought Co. Last modified February 16, 2019. ThoughtCo.com /bell-hooks-biography-3530371.

Jones, Ida E. "Mary McLeod Bethune, True Democracy, and the Fight for Universal Suffrage." National Park Service. Last modified December 14, 2020. NPS.gov /articles/000/mary-mcleod-bethune-true-democracy -and-the-fight-for-universal-suffrage.htm.

Lange, Allison. "National Women's Party and Militant Methods." National Women's History Museum, 2015. CrusadeForTheVote.org/nwp-militant.

Lange, Allison. "Suffragists Organize: American Woman Suffrage Association." National Women's History Museum, 2015. CrusadeForTheVote.org/ awsa-organize.

Library of Congress. "Historical Overview of the National Women's Party." Accessed February 17, 2021. LOC.gov /static/collections/women-of-protest/images /history.pdf.

Matias, Dani. "New Report Says Women Will Soon Be Majority of College-Educated U.S. Workers." NPR. June 20, 2019. NPR.org/2019/06/20/734408574 /new-report-says-college-educated-women-will-soon -make-up-majority-of-u-s-labor-f.

Michals, Debra. "Alice Paul." National Women's History Museum, 2015. WomensHistory.org/education -resources/biographies/alice-paul.

Michals, Debra. "Betty Friedan." National Women's History Museum, 2017. WomensHistory.org /education-resources/biographies/betty-friedan.

Michals, Debra. "Elizabeth Cady Stanton." National Women's History Museum, 2017. WomensHistory.org /education-resources/biographies/elizabeth-cady -stanton.

Michals, Debra. "Gloria Steinem." National Women's History Museum, 2017. WomensHistory.org /education-resources/biographies/gloria-steinem.

Michals, Debra. "Mary McLeod Bethune." National Women's History Museum, 2015. WomensHistory.org /education-resources/biographies/mary-mcleod -bethune.

Michals, Debra. "Sojourner Truth." National Women's History Museum, 2015. WomensHistory.org/education -resources/biographies/sojourner-truth.

National Museum of American History. "Who Was Left Out of the Story?" Accessed February 22, 2021. AmericanHistory.si.edu/creating-icons/who-was-left-out-story.

National Park Service. "Dr. Mabel Ping-Hua Lee." Accessed February 23, 2021. NPS.gov/people/mabel-lee.htm.

National Park Service. "Elizabeth Cady Stanton." Accessed February 20, 2021. NPS.gov/wori/learn/historyculture/elizabeth-cady-stanton.htm.

National Park Service. "Marie Louise Bottineau Baldwin." Accessed February 22, 2021. NPS.gov/people/marie-louise-bottineau-baldwin.htm.

National Park Service. "Mary McLeod Bethune." Accessed February 22, 2021. NPS.gov/mamc/learn/historyculture/mary-mcleod-bethune.htm.

National Park Service. "Nina Otero-Warren." Accessed February 22, 2021. NPS.gov/people/nina-otero-warren.htm.

National Susan B. Anthony Museum & House. "Her Life." Accessed February 20, 2021. SusanB.org/her-life.

New Mexico Historic Women Marker Initiative. "Nina Otero-Warren." Accessed February 22, 2021. NMHistoricWomen.org/location/nina-otero-warren.

Norwood, Arlisha R. "Ida B. Wells-Barnett." National Women's History Museum, 2017. WomensHistory.org /education-resources/biographies/ida-b-wells-barnett.

Office of Gloria Steinem. "Gloria Steinem." Accessed February 26, 2021. GloriaSteinem.com/about.

Parkinson, Hilary. "19th Amendment at 100: Mabel Ping-Hua Lee." US National Archives. May 5, 2020. prologue.blogs.archives.gov/2020/05/05/19th -amendment-at-100-mabel-ping-hua-lee.

Parkinson, Hilary. "19th Amendment at 100: Mary Louise Bottineau Baldwin." US National Archives. April 2, 2020. prologue.blogs.archives.gov/2020/04/02/19th -amendment-at-100-mary-louise-bottineau-baldwin.

Redman, Henry. "List Maintenance or Voter Purges: How the Practice Of Maintaining Voter Lists Become So Polarized." *Microsoft News.* October 9, 2020. MSN.com/en-us/news/politics/list-maintenance -or-voter-purges-how-the-practice-of-maintaining -voter-lists-become-so-polarized/ar-BB19RkeG.

Shteir, Rachel. "Why We Can't Stop Talking about Betty Friedan." *The New York Times.* February 3, 2021. NYTimes.com/2021/02/03/us/betty-friedan -feminism-legacy.html.

Sojourner Truth Memorial Committee. "Her Story." Sojourner Truth Memorial. Accessed February 18, 2021. SojournerTruthMemorial.org/sojourner-truth /her-history.

Stacey Abrams for Governor. "Meet Stacey." Accessed February 26, 2021. StaceyAbrams.com/meet-stacey.

About the Author

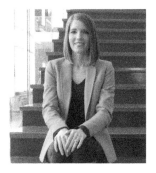

Meghan Vestal is a former teacher and the founder of the curriculum development company Vestal's 21st Century Classroom LLC. She has created hands-on curricula for thousands of teachers and schools around the world and designed unique professional development opportunities for teachers. Her educational programs have been recognized by the US Congress. She is also the author of *Geology for Kids: A Junior Scientist's Guide to Rocks, Minerals, and the Earth Beneath Our Feet*.

You can learn more about Meghan by visiting Vestal's 21st Century Classroom's website or YouTube channel.

About the Illustrator

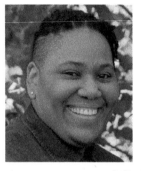 **Keisha Morris** grew up in Charlottesville, Virginia, and currently resides in Maryland. She spends her days creating stories and developing characters that inspire, bring joy, and promote wonder. She creates her illustrations by collaging tissue paper and finishing her illustrations in Photoshop. This allows her to produce whimsical, vibrant, and eye-catching illustrations that ignite the imagination. In her free time, Keisha enjoys spending time with her wife, daughter, and two crazy cats, Ollie and Elphie (named after Elphaba from Gregory Maguire's *Wicked*, and yes, she is a black cat!). She also enjoys traveling, watching reruns of *Buffy the Vampire Slayer*, animated movies, listening to podcasts, and weight lifting.